Biomaterials in Hand Surgery

Antonio Merolli · Thomas J. Joyce (Eds.)

Biomaterials in Hand Surgery

Foreword by
Frédéric Schuind

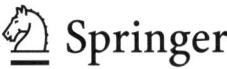 Springer

Editors
Antonio Merolli
Orthopaedics and Hand Surgery
The Catholic University School of Medicine
Rome
Italy

Thomas J. Joyce
School of Mechanical and Systems Engineering
Newcastle University
Newcastle upon Tyne
United Kingdom

ISBN 978-88-470-1194-6   e-ISBN 978-88-470-1195-3

DOI 10.1007/978-88-470-1195-3

Springer Dordrecht Heidelberg London Milan New York

Library of Congress Control Number: 2009920945

© Springer Verlag Italia 2009

Typesetting: Graphostudio, Milan, Italy
Printing and binding: Arti Grafiche Nidasio, Assago (MI), Italy
Printed in Italy

Springer-Verlag Italia S.r.l. – Via Decembrio 28 – I-20137 Milan
Springer is a part of Springer Science+Business Media (www.springer.com)

Foreword

Biomaterials are used in many areas of medicine, particularly in surgery and dentistry. In orthopedic surgery, total hip arthroplasty has been extremely successful, and has been called 'the operation of the 20th century'. Total hip arthroplasty is routinely performed every day in most orthopedic departments. Over the last decades, many efforts have been made to better integrate the components within the recipient bones, to decrease the friction at the prosthetic interface, and to minimize wear. Minimally invasive procedures have been developed, and various designs are intended to preserve as much as possible of the bone stock of young patients. By contrast, the clinical results have been less favorable after various hand and wrist joint replacements. Many early designs have failed, the clinical data of the current prostheses are frequently quite limited, and there is often insufficient biomechanical information available, although trapezio-metacarpal arthroplasty in particular has become quite popular in recent years. In order to promote progress in hand and wrist arthroplasty, Antonio Merolli and Thomas J. Joyce have edited this lovely book, whose chapters discuss current research and recent advances in hand and wrist arthroplasty. The problems of metacarpophalangeal joint prostheses are particularly developed.

Biomaterials have many other potential applications in hand surgery. New fixation designs are low profile and stable, yet allow immediate postoperative motion, which is so important for rapid and total recovery of hand function. Coated implants could be used in contaminated situations. Biodegradable osteosynthesis implants, although currently disappointing, will possibly be improved in the coming years, especially for use in the hand and wrist. The hand surgeon is also faced with devastating traumas, where tissue engineering could in the future be the solution to replace various tissues. As discussed in the book, biomaterial coating of flexor tendon sutures could improve tendon gliding. Novel biomaterials could also very soon replace nerve autografts, which are of limited supply and require additional surgery for harvesting; they could possibly also enhance axonal regeneration. This book, the first to my knowledge devoted to biomaterials in hand surgery, is, therefore, recommended as required reading for those interested in advances in hand reconstruction, whether undergraduate medical or engineering students or consultants in hand surgery, rheumatologists or material scientists.

Brussels, June 2009   **Frédéric Schuind, MD, PhD**
Department of Orthopaedics and Traumatology
Erasme University Hospital
Brussels, Belgium

Preface

This book is the first devoted to the application of biomaterials in hand surgery. It presents the fundamentals of biomaterials, tissue engineering and regenerative medicine, the finite elements method, and hand joint prostheses. It examines in depth the key topic of metacarpophalangeal joint prostheses in rheumatoid patients. In addition, it reviews the trends in tendon research and peripheral nerve regeneration with artificial nerve guides.

Several topics are current fields of research and debate, so they have been informed by the personal experience of the contributing authors; they do not intend to give the definitive solution for a problem but instead propose a way to reach such a resolution.

Our main purpose is to gather information in the field of biomaterials in hand surgery in a single dedicated book that can be accessed by readers with different levels of knowledge (from undergraduate medical or engineering students to consultants in hand surgery) and different specialized interests (for example: clinicians caring for rheumatoid patients, or material scientists wishing to improve their knowledge about peripheral nerve regeneration).

The authors are aware that it is possible some topics may have been neglected or overlooked; for others, progress is very fast and new data have accumulated while the book was being produced; for these reasons the contributors will be happy to receive comments and suggestions for improving and updating this book. Together we hope you will help us to create a reference text for the field of biomaterials in hand surgery.

Antonio Merolli
Thomas J. Joyce

Contents

6 Prosthetic Surgery of Metacarpophalangeal Joints in Rheumatoid Patients:
an Open Problem
Francesco Catalano

7 Requirements for a Metacarpophalangeal Joint Prosthesis for Rheumatoid
Patients and Suggestions for Design
Antonio Merolli

8 Research Trends for Flexor Tendon Repair
Stavros Thomopoulos

9 Peripheral Nerve Regeneration by Artificial Nerve Guides
Antonio Merolli and Lorenzo Rocchi

List of Contributors

Luigi Ambrosio
Institute for Composite and
Biomedical Materials
National Research Council
Naples, Italy

Francesco Catalano
Orthopaedics and Hand Surgery
The Catholic University School
of Medicine
Rome, Italy

Thomas J. Joyce
School of Mechanical and
Systems Engineering
Newcastle University
Newcastle upon Tyne
United Kingdom

Antonio Merolli
Orthopaedics and Hand Surgery
The Catholic University School
of Medicine
Rome, Italy

Francesco Mollica
Department of Engineering
University of Ferrara
Ferrara, Italy

Lorenzo Rocchi
Orthopaedics and Hand Surgery
The Catholic University School
of Medicine
Rome, Italy

Matteo Santin
Pharmacy and Biomolecular Sciences
University of Brighton
Brighton, United Kingdom

Stavros Thomopoulos
Orthopedic Surgery and
Biomedical Engineering
Washington University
St. Louis, MO, USA

Paolo Tranquilli Leali
Orthopaedic Surgery
University of Sassari
Sassari, Italy

Abbreviations

bFGF	basic fibroblast growth factor
BMP	bone morphogenetic protein
BSEM	back-scattered electron microscopy
CAD	computer-aided/assisted design
CAE	computer-aided/assisted engineering
CAM	computer-aided/assisted manufacturing
cd-HA	carbodiimide derivatized hyaluronic acid
CMC-I	carpal-metacarpal joint I
CNS	central nervous system
CT	computerized tomography
2D	two-dimensional
3D	three-dimensional
DIP	distal interphalangeal (joint)
ECM	extracellular matrix
EGF	epidermal growth factor
ESC	embryonic stem cell
FEM	finite element method
FGF	fibroblast growth factor
GAG	glycosaminoglycan
HA	hyaluronic acid/hyaluronan
HA	hydroxyapatite
hESC	human embryonic stem cell
HSC	hematopoietic stem cell
IGF	insulin-like growth factor
iPSC	induced pluripotent stem cell
IVF	*in vitro* fertilization
MCP	metacarpophalangeal (joint)
MSC	mesenchymal stem cell
NGF	nerve growth factor
PCM	pericellular matrix

PDGF	platelet-derived growth factor
PE	polyethylene
PEG	polyethylene glycol
PGN	proteoglycan
PIP	proximal interphalangeal (joint)
PLA	poly-L-lactic acid
PMMA	polymethyl-methacrylate
RA	rheumatoid arthritis
TGF	transforming growth factor
TMC	trapezio-metacarpal (joint)
VEGF	vascular endothelial growth factor

Fundamentals of Biomaterials 1

P. Tranquilli Leali and A. Merolli

Abstract The definition for "biomaterial" proposed by the *European Society for Biomaterials Consensus Conference II* quotes: "A biomaterial is a material intended to interface with biological systems to evaluate, treat, augment or replace any tissue, organ or function of the body". In hand surgery, biomaterials may interact with tendons, nerves, and bones. Interaction with bone is, by far, the most often required, and the vast amount of knowledge accumulated in relation to other anatomic regions, such as the hip or knee, can be transferred to the hand. This chapter reviews the main classes of materials that may be used in hand surgery, with an emphasis on what has been acquired by histomorphological studies.

Keywords Biomaterial • Ceramics • Composites • Hand Surgery • Metals • Polymers

1.1
Introduction

The term "biomaterial" seems to be in a continuous evolution, but we can rely on the definition proposed by the *European Society for Biomaterials Consensus Conference II*: "A biomaterial is a material intended to interface with biological systems to evaluate, treat, augment or replace any tissue, organ or function of the body" [1].

Generally, biomaterials are divided into classes, according to their material properties, so we have metals, polymers, ceramics, etc. But they can be also categorized according to the response they elicit from living tissues, so we have biologically inert materials, bioactive materials, biomimetic materials, etc.

In hand surgery, biomaterials may interact with tendons, nerves, and bones. Interaction with bone is, by far, the most often required, and the vast amount of knowledge accumulated in other anatomic regions, such as the hip or knee, can be transferred to the hand.

Morphology gives important clues in characterizing the interaction with bone, and the two techniques of choice for the analysis of the bone–biomaterial interface are polarized light miscroscopy and back-scattered electron microscopy (BSEM). The technique of BSEM is particularly appropriate for study of the interface between bone and biomaterials because it allows picturing of a map of material distribution where

P. Tranquilli Leali (✉)
Orthopaedics Surgery, University of Sassari, Sassari, Italy

A. Merolli, T.J. Joyce (eds), *Biomaterials in Hand Surgery.*
© Springer-Verlag Italia 2009

implanted materials with different densities, bone tissue in different stages of maturation, embedding media, and artifactual cracks are easily discernible (Fig. 1.1). With this technique, electrons are directed at a certain angle towards the surface of the sample and interact with the material so they are reflected with a different energy; the final energy is detected and rendered in a graphic form by a gray tone [2] on a photomicrograph.

With this perspective, we basically have two classes of materials: (a) materials promoting a tight apposition of newly formed bone; and (b) materials not promoting a tight apposition of newly formed bone. The morphological character of tight apposition is present whenever osteocytes may be found within a few micrometers of the material, and the newly formed bone, which they produced, interlocks with the material so

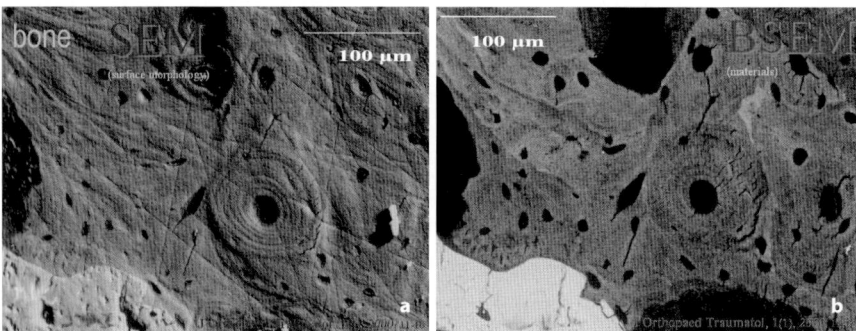

Fig. 1.1 A sample of hydroxyapatite-coated metallic substrate implanted in bone, when analyzed by scanning electron microscopy (**a**), allows evaluation of topographical characters such as: the alignment of lamellae, the location of Haversian systems, the porosity of the hydroxyapatite coating. Then, if on the same field of observation, a back-scattered electron microscopy analysis follows (**b**), it is possible to evaluate the actual material distribution on the sample and clearly discern metallic substrate; hydoxyapatite coating; bone tissue in different stages of maturation; embedding media and artefactual detachments. Reproduced with permission from [2]

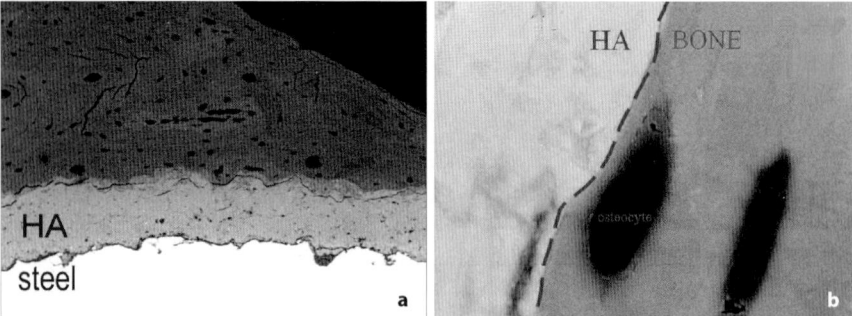

Fig. 1.2 The morphological character of tight appositionis present whenever osteocytes are found within a few micrometers of the material, and the newly formed bone, which they produced, interlocks with the material so tightly that even a high-magnification electron microscopic analysis cannot resolve any discontinuity at the interface. **a**, reproduced with permission from [3]; **b**, reproduced with permission from [2]. *HA*, hydroxyapatite

tightly that even high-magnification electron microscopic analysis cannot resolve any discontinuity at the interface [2]. Bioactive ceramics like hydroxyapatite and bioactive glass (see later) typically elicit this type of bone response and they are often used as coatings for devices manufactured with materials that are unable to induce tight apposition, to promote a similar response towards them (Fig. 1.2) [2, 3].

Next, we will review the main classes of materials that may be used in hand surgery.

1.2
Metals

Stainless steel, cobalt chrome, and titanium alloys are widely used because of their mechanical strength [4]. They are key materials in devices needed for osteosynthesis, in which they must guarantee mechanical stability in the early phases of fracture healing, prior to completion of the healing process.

Designing a metallic device generally achieves the goal of coping with the mechanical performance that is required. Problems may arise from the biological response at the metal–bone interface (Fig. 1.3); several stainless steel alloys promote a fibrous reaction that may result in a multicellular layer of fibroblasts interposed between the recipient bone and the implant, eventually leading to implant loosening. Titanium alloys are better able to promote an integration with bone and, sometimes, only a tiny non-ossified rim remains between them and the recipient bone, so thin that it can only be recognized by the higher magnification provided by electron microscopy.

A range of surface treatments has been developed and applied to metallic implants to better integrate with the recipient bone or, even, to mask the metal to the bone by a variety of processes that can be grouped under the term of "biomimicry". A hydroxyapatite coating is the most widely applied biomimetic treatment for metallic surfaces; several other methods have been proposed, some of which have reached clinical application, such as bioactive glass coating or anodic oxidation.

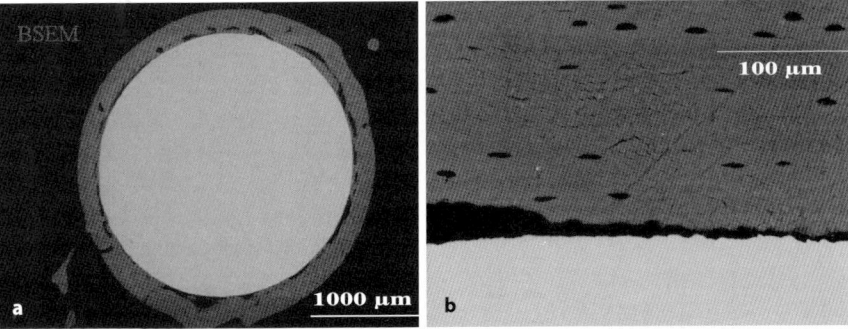

Fig. 1.3 Even when newly formed bone can be found growing around a metallic implant (**a**), a higher magnification analysis by electron microscopy may identify a tiny non-ossified rim which remains between bone and metal (**b**). Reproduced with permission from [3]

1.3
Polymers

Several classes of polymers interact with bone tissue in applications where they are required as artifacts to be put in direct apposition with bone or as eventual wear products of artifacts implanted in skeletal structures.

To study the characteristics of bone tissue response to medical polymers, in a comparative way, the choice of a well-defined animal model is fundamental. In the past, the distal meta-epiphyseal region of the femur in New Zealand White rabbits has often been used. Here, the presence of abundant trabecular bone helps in describing the character of bone response in terms of both time and quantity.

Highlighting the morphological response at the interface between bone and various kinds of polymers, a common general pattern can be recognized that can be described as a "confinement reaction", where bone tissue grows, matures, and remodels around the polymeric implant. Experiments with unloaded implants show that in the absence of inflammatory foreign-body reactions to wear debris, polymers such as polyethylene, poly-L-lactic acid (PLA) (Fig. 1.4), polyetherimide, etc, comply with the physiologic turnover and remodeling of surrounding bone, leading to the morphological picture of a bony rim that encloses the implant.

When long-term implantation is studied, bone tissue shows the characteristics of corticalization, which means that it is likely to create a new outer border in its structure (Fig. 1.5) [5].

What is not elicited by the most commonly used medical polymers is some kind of bioactivity or biomimicry, as occurs with bioceramic materials like hydroxyapatite or bioactive glass (see later). This limitation led to the development of the field of polymeric–bioactive materials composites (PLA–bioactive glass or polyethylene (PE)–hydroxyapatite, for example) which, then, can be considered a new class of biomaterials (see later).

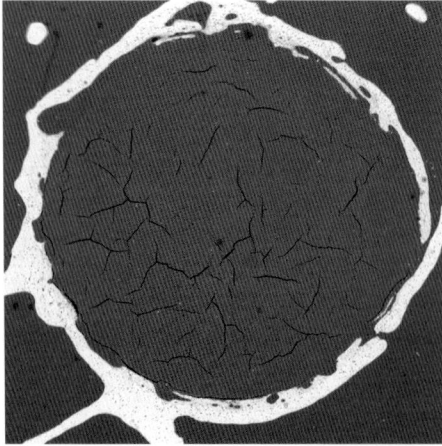

Fig. 1.4 The character of bone response to polymers can be described as a "confinement reaction". In this BSEM cross-section, bone has grown all around a cylinder of poly-L-lactic acid, whose presence after 12 months of implantation can be inferred by the cracks produced from heating of the material by the electron beam

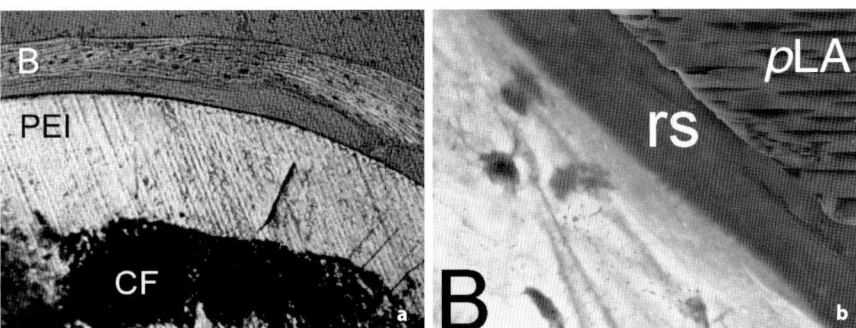

Fig. 1.5 Bone response to polymers. **a** Polarized light microscopic analysis shows an outer border of bone (*B*) which surronds a polyetherimide (*PEI*) cylinder filled with carbon fibers (*CF*) (reproduced with permission from [5]). **b** BSEM shows that there is a space which separates bone (*B*) from poly-L-lactic acid (*pLA*), as evidenced by a rim of embedding resin (*rs*) in between; the heating of the electron beam affects poly-L-lactic acid more quickly than the embedding resin

1.3.1
Polymethyl-methacrylate

Polymethyl-methacrylate (PMMA) has become the material of choice for attaching an implant to bone, for example cementing the stem of a joint prosthesis to the host bone. PMMA has probably been overused, in the sense that sometimes the cement has been required to cope with the mechanical mismatch between the implant and the recipient bone: for example, when stability is needed for a stem subjected to torsion, or when an osteoporotic bone, too weak to bear the load transmitted at a joint, receives an implant. Fracture of the cement, and debris production, which may occur in these cases, have been considered in the past more a cause than a consequence of the mechanical mismatch, prompting the possible avoidance of the use of PMMA cement (as in cementless joint prostheses).

From the surgical point of view, the easy intraoperative workability of PMMA cement favored several other applications apart from cementing joint stems, such as filling the large bone cavities produced by the surgical removal of a tumor; in this application, PMMA often assured a long-lasting mechanical stability and compatibility with the recipient bone [6].

Furthermore, PMMA has been applied as an *in situ* drug-delivery system for antibiotics in cavities produced by osteomyelytis [7]. It has also been proposed as a drug-delivery system for antiblastic drugs in the *in situ* therapy of tumors affecting bone [8].

More recently, PMMA has been used as a moldable material to cast temporary spacers after the removal of failed joint prostheses that were involved in an infectious process; in this case, PMMA is not required to provide any mechanical performance but simply to give a provisional congruence to the joint ends, for the time required by drug therapy to control and hopefully eradicate the infection and, then, allow implantation of a revision prosthesis.

1.3.2
Polyethylene

PE experienced great success in the past because it was easily formed into many different shapes and seemed to be an ideal counterface in the coupling with a metallic component in artificial joints. However, it is now recognized that PE wear debris can provoke a negative cascade of reactions within the body that can cause osteolysis and loosening of the implant. The search for a lower-wearing PE was pursued by a constant increase in molecular weight and, recently, by optimizing the cross-linking of the chains.

PE has been proposed as a material for temporary multiple-sized joint spacers following the removal of infected artificial joints, but its main application today remains in coupling with the metallic component of an artificial joint, such as, for example, facing the mirror-finished metallic condyles with an articular plate in the interphalangeal joint [9].

1.3.3
Biodegradable Polymers

Performing osteosynthesis with the implantation of a metallic device inside the body sometimes promotes development of an infectious process that, in the past, has even led to amputation of the infected limb. Infection can arise a long time after the end of the healing process, so, bearing this in mind, mantaining a metallic device for a longer time, or even for life, is not recommended.

However, the rule of removing an osteosynthesis device after completion of the healing process (and, generally, not longer than 12 months from implantation) is not easy to implement for two main reasons: the first is that in several parts of the body the second operation required to remove the implant may be difficult and risky; the second is that it is costly.

The idea of having devices made of biodegradable polymers that were able to sustain the mechanical load during the healing process of a fracture but, afterwards, would gradually disappear from the site, was greeted with great enthusiasm in the early 1990s (Fig. 1.6).

To summarize the long story of biodegradable materials in orthopedic surgery [10], the following observations can be made: (a) the mechanical properties of the metallic devices that were to be substituted were seldom matched by the proposed biodegradable materials; (b) the operative techniques with these materials required greater care and, in some ways, a different attitude in the sense that great care had to be taken not to break the implant (while with metallic devices the emphasis was more on "not breaking the bone").

Reduction in costs, which could be obtained by avoiding a second operation for removal, was hampered by the significantly higher cost of biodegradable implants. But the biggest disappointment came from the discrepancy that exists between the biological and clinical acception of "degradation". In fact, several devices made from

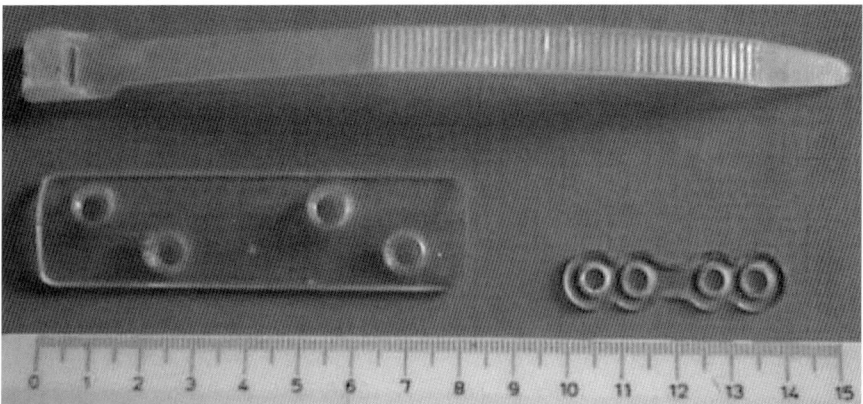

Fig. 1.6 The idea of having devices made of biodegradable polymers which were able to sustain the mechanical load during the healing process of a fracture but, afterwards, would gradually disappear from the site, was greeted with great enthusiasm in the early 1990s, when authors developed and tested new plates and bands made of with different blends of poly-L-lactic acid

biodegradable polymers did not perform clinically as "degradable" because of their long degradation time *in vivo* [11].

There is a discrepancy between what is "degradable" from a chemical point of view and what can be considered "degradable" from a clinical point of view. Materials science can describe the degradable behavior of a material on the basis of its chemical properties. Often, a direct cellular contribution, for example in the form of enzymatic digestion, can further characterize the degradation properties of a material and, in this case, the term "bioresorption" may be more appropriate. In any case, "degradation" or "resorption" of a material and of a device should not be considered in terms of the actual time needed for the *in vitro* or *in vivo* processes to occur, but should be correlated with the time required by the healing process in which the material and device interact. After healing has been accomplished, the degradable implant is no longer needed and could even behave as an unwanted cause of a bone defect.

Biodegradable implants proposed in hand surgery are made mostly of PLA blends and have selected applications. An ever-increasing number of designs has been developed for lightly loaded, small implants.

1.4
Ceramics

Inert non-bioactive ceramics, like alumina (Al_2O_3), are used in clinical practice as bearings in total joint replacements, because of their resistance to wear and their positive tribological properties [12]. Alumina–PE prostheses have been proposed for interphalangeal and metacarpophalangeal joint prostheses [13]. However, they can be expensive, and concerns over the potential of fracture remain.

Bioactive ceramics are employed as coatings to enhance the fixation of a device, or as bone-graft substitutes because of their osteoconductive properties. They act as a scaffold to enhance bone formation on their surface.

1.4.1
Hydroxyapatite

Hydroxyapatite is the most widely used bioactive ceramic material in surgery.

Bone may be defined as a composite tissue with an organic matrix composed primarily of the protein collagen, which provides flexibility (about 10% of adult bone mass is collagen), and a mineral phase that is composed of hydroxyapatite, which is an insoluble salt of calcium and phosphorus (about 65% of adult bone mass is hydroxyapatite); water comprises approximately 25% of adult bone mass. It is the collagen fibers and calcium salts that help to strengthen bone. In fact, the collagen fibers of bone have great tensile strength, while the calcium salts have great compressive strength. These combined properties, plus the degree of bondage between the collagen fibers and the crystals, provide a bony structure that has extreme tensile and compressive strength.

The discovery that osteoblasts can grow happily on artificial hydroxyapatite, both as a bulk material and as a plasma-spray coating, improved significantly the possibility of obtaining a favorable response to the implantation of devices that were loaded or coated with industrial-made hydroxyapatite (Fig. 1.7a) [14].

Not only are osteoblasts found growing on hydroxyapatite, but osteoclasts also seem able to remove it (Fig. 1.7b), in this way reproducing the physiological "turnover" process of apposition and removal that occurs in living bone [14].

This property well deserves the name of "biomimicry" [15], and coating an implant with hydroxyapatite became an effective system to mask the structural material that it

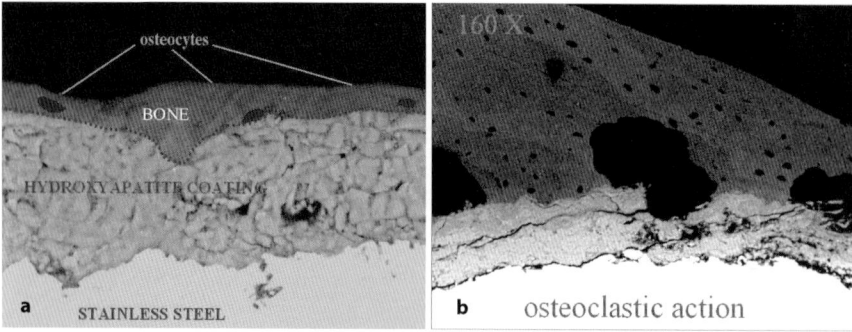

Fig. 1.7 Osteoblasts can grow on artificial hydroxyapatite coating, improving significantly the possibility of obtaining a favorable response towards a coated metallic devices (**a**) (reproduced with permission from [14]). Traces of an osteoclast "byte", removing bone and hydroxyapatite coating as well, suggest that the physiologic "turnover" process of apposition and removal can occur on a hydroxyapatite-coated implant (**b**). Reproduced with permission from [2]

is made of, promoting an early favorable response from recipient bone towards the implant.

Hydroxyapatite is also used as bone filler when large cavities are encountered. It must be underlined that, in this role, complete resorption of the material is not always obtained, even in the long term; furthermore, hydroxyapatite can be used as a filler only when no real mechanical task is required.

1.4.2
Bioactive Glass

In the 1970s, Professor Larry Hench discovered that a particular range of glass composition could elicit favorable growth of bone cells [16]. A particular application in orthopedic surgery came from the deposition of a bioactive glass coating (Fig. 1.8) in a similar fashion to a hydroxyapatite coating [17].

The rationale for a degradable bioactive glass coating is to lead the bone to appose gradually to the metal without the production of bulky non-degradable particles, such as those observed with fragmentation of the crystalline phase of hydroxyapatite coatings [18].

Since the development of the first bioactive glass by Hench, several kinds of glass and glass-ceramics have been found to interface with living bone. The model in this class of materials is Bioglass 45S5, whose composition by weight is: 45% SiO_2, 24.5% CaO, 6% P_2O_5, and 24.5% Na_2O. The bonding mechanism of silicate bioactive glass to bone has been attributed to a series of surface reactions that ultimately lead to the formation of a hydroxycarbonate apatite layer at the glass surface. The critical element necessary for formation of this layer is the production of a porous silica gel with a high surface area. The apatite phase is formed when the bioactive material comes into contact with the aqueous component of physiologic fluids.

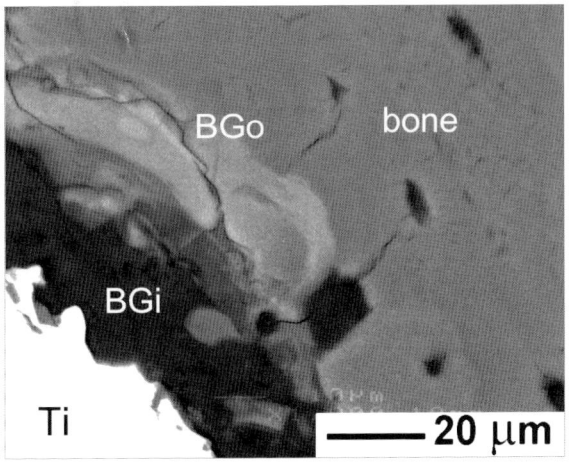

Fig. 1.8 A bioactive glass coating of titanium alloy (*Ti*) may elicit a tight apposition of newly formed bone. The bioactive glass coating gradually increases its concentration of calcium ions, as evidenced by this BSEM where a less calcified inner layer (*BGi*) can be differentiated from a more calcified outer layer (*BGo*). The interface between glass and bone is virtually indistinguishable

Standardization of hydroxyapatite coating techniques for orthopedic implants has, probably, limited the exploitation of bioactive glass coatings in orthopedic surgery, while it is applied more in dental and maxillo-facial surgery.

1.5
Composites

Composite materials made from carbon fibers and epoxide resins were proposed to replace metals. This replacement process occurred in other fields, such as the aerospace industry, but in orthopedic surgery the possible unmasking of carbon fibers, and their dispersion inside the body, were unacceptable risks. High cost was another important concern.

Nevertheless, attempts are being made to find a place for composites in bone surgery in other preparations [19]. The two most common families of composites proposed are: (a) biodegradable material–ceramics (or glass) composite [20,21]; and (b) PE–hydroxyapatite [22].

Composites between a biodegradable polymer and a ceramic or a glass material have been developed, with the aim of taking advantage of the degradability of the polymer while trying to avoid any excessive inflammatory reaction towards its breakdown products as a result of the bioceramic component, which should also help in the early stages of interaction with bone.

The same principle applies to the PE–hydroxyapatite composite: this material has already been applied in the clinic, in fields like inner-ear surgery. Applications are envisaged for small implants, such as those required in hand surgery.

References

1. Doherty PJ, Williams RL, Williams DF, Lee JC (eds) (1992) Biomaterial–Tissue Interfaces, Advances in Biomaterials, 10. Elsevier, Amsterdam.
2. Merolli A, Tranquilli Leali, De Santis E (2000) A back-scattered electron microscopy (BSEM) study of the tight apposition between bone and hydroxyapatite coating. J Orthopaed Traumatol 1:11–16.
3. Merolli A, Moroni A, Faldini C et al (2003) Histomorphological study of bone response to hydroxyapatite coating on stainless steel. J Mater Sci Mater Med 14:327–333.
4. Niinomi M (2008) Metallic biomaterials. J Artif Organs 11:105–110.
5. Merolli A, Perrone V, Tranquilli Leali P (1999) Response to polyetherimide based composite materials implanted in muscle and in bone. J Mater Sci Mater Med 10:265–268.
6. Aboulafia AJ, Levine AM, Schmidt D, Aboulafia D (2007) Surgical therapy of bone metastases. Semin Oncol 34:206–214.
7. Kent ME, Rapp RP, Smith KM (2006) Antibiotic beads and osteomyelitis: here today, what's coming tomorrow? Orthopedics 29:599–603.
8. Greco F, de Palma L, Specchia N et al (1992) Polymethylmethacrylate-antiblastic drug compounds: an in vitro study assessing the cytotoxic effect in cancer cell lines-a new method for local chemotherapy of bone metastasis. Orthopedics 15:189–194.

9. Ash HE, Unsworth A (2000) Design of a surface replacement prosthesis for the proximal interphalangeal joint. Proc Inst Mech Eng 214:151–163.
10. Middleton JC, Tipton AJ (2000) Synthetic biodegradable polymers as orthopedic devices. Biomaterials 21:2335–2346.
11. Merolli A, Gabbi C, Cacchioni A et al (2001) Bone response to polymers based on poly-lactic acid and having different degradation times. J Mater Sci Mater Med 12:775–778.
12. Hamadouche M, Sedel L (2000) Ceramics in orthopaedics. J Bone Joint Surg Br 82B:1095–1099.
13. Doi K, Kuwata N, Kawai S (1984) Alumina ceramic finger implants: a preliminary biomaterial and clinical evaluation. J Hand Surg (Am) 9:740–749.
14. Tranquilli Leali P, Merolli A, Palmacci O et al (1994) Evaluation of different preparations of plasma-spray hydroxyapatite coating on titanium alloy and duplex stainless steel in the rabbit. J Mater Sci Mater Med 5:345–349.
15. Williams D (1995) Biomimetic surfaces: how man-made becomes man-like. Med Device Technol 6:6–8.
16. Hench LL, Splinter RJ, Allen WC, Greenlee TK (1971) Bonding mechanisms at the interface of ceramic prosthetic materials. J Biomed Mater Res 2:117–121.
17. Merolli A, Guidi PL, Gianotta L, Tranquilli Leali P (1999) The clinical outcome of bioactive glass coated hip prostheses. In: Ohgushi H, Hastings GW, Yoshikawa T (eds) Bioceramics 12. World Scientific, Singapore, pp 597–600.
18. Merolli A, Gabbi C, Santin M et al (2004) Bioactive glass coatings on Ti6Al4V promote the tight apposition of newly-formed bone in-vivo. Key Eng Materials 254–256:789–792.
19. Stein PS, Sullivan J, Haubenreich JE, Osborne PB (2005) Composite resin in medicine and dentistry. J Long Term Eff Med Implants 15:641–654.
20. Boeree NR, Dove J, Cooper JJ et al (1993) Development of a degradable composite for orthopaedic use: mechanical evaluation of an hydroxyapatite-polyhydroxybutyrate composite material. Biomaterials 14:793–796.
21. Närhi TO, Jansen JA, Jaakkola T et al (2003) Bone response to degradable thermoplastic composite in rabbits. Biomaterials 24:1697–1704.
22. Di Silvio L, Dalby M, Bonfield W (1998) In vitro response of osteoblasts to hydroxyapatite-reinforced polyethylene composites. J Mater Sci Mater Med 9:845–848.

Potential Applications of Tissue Engineering in Hand Surgery

2

M. Santin

Abstract Tissue engineering is a relatively new discipline aiming at the regeneration of tissues and organs that have been damaged by either traumatic events or diseases. From a technological viewpoint, tissue regeneration is pursued by implantation of the so-called tissue engineering constructs. A tissue engineering construct is based on 3D biomaterials that are able to host and deliver cell types relevant to the regeneration of the target tissue. Ideally, biomaterials should also be able to control the behavior of cells, directing their ability to synthesize and deposit new tissue components. This property should either be intrinsically built into the biomaterial 3D scaffold or achieved through integration of bioactive molecules such as growth factors and drugs. Also, in some clinical scenarios, the possibility of delivering the tissue engineering construct as an injectable formulation should be considered, to facilitate minimally invasive surgery. In this chapter, the main biomaterials and engineering methods for obtaining 3D scaffolds will be presented, together with an overview of the most recommended cell types, the stem cells. A review of specific factors and bioactive molecules that can be included to improve the tissue regeneration potential of the tissue engineering construct is also provided. Finally, the potential of tissue engineering to treat tissues relevant to hand surgery is presented, and the clinical applicability is critically assessed.

Keywords Bioactive Molecules • Biodegradable Biomaterials • Growth Factors • Stem Cells • Tissue Engineering • Tissue Repair

2.1
Introduction

Hand surgery presents a challenge to the surgeon as complex procedures are required to simultaneously repair several types of tissues. Fractured or diseased bones, degraded cartilage, severed tendons and nerves, as well as traumatized muscles and skin may be damaged beyond their ability to self-repair and, as a consequence, they need surgical procedures that can promote their healing. Currently, these surgical approaches are

M. Santin (✉)
Pharmacy and Biomolecular Sciences, University of Brighton, Brighton, United Kingdom

A. Merolli, T.J. Joyce (eds), *Biomaterials in Hand Surgery.*
© Springer-Verlag Italia 2009

based on reconstructive procedures in which biomedical implants play an important part (e.g. finger prostheses, metal plates, neural guides) [1].

2.1.1
Limitations of Permanent Implants

In surgical procedures, biomedical implants based on polymeric, metallic and ceramic biomaterials exert their role by replacing the structure and biomechanics of the damaged tissue. With the exception of biodegradable suturing materials and some of the commercially available neural guides [2, 3], most of these implants are non-degradable and they are implanted with the goal of replacing the damaged tissue rather than repairing/regenerating it.

While partially restoring the biomechanical and aesthetic features of the damaged tissue, these devices have a limited ability to integrate within the damaged tissue as well as with other surrounding anatomical components and, as a consequence, their life span is relatively short [4]. In particular, these non-degradable biomaterials do not allow the implant to participate in the later tissue remodeling, and often they are not able to translate the mechanical loads appropriately to the surrounding tissue. These limitations often have a negative impact on the clinical outcome of the hand reconstruction process.

2.1.2
Biodegradable Biomaterials: from Tissue Replacement to Tissue Regeneration

In the last few decades, bioresorbable/biodegradable biomaterials have been widely investigated in an attempt to achieve complete tissue repair in surgery [5]. Rather than focusing on replacement of the damaged tissue by permanent devices, the gradual degradation of these materials has the potential to accompany the formation of new tissue. As mentioned before, hand surgery has exploited biodegradable biomaterials to obtain mainly soft tissue healing; suturing and neural guides for peripheral nerve regeneration are typical examples of biodegradable biomaterials employed in this clinical application [2, 3]. These biodegradable biomaterials play a role as a physical support for the repairing tissue and they do not actively participate in its biochemical and cellular processes. Furthermore, no clinical solution has yet been designed to jump-start the repair/regeneration of bone and tendons in those cases where the extent of damage or the presence of a pathology impairs the endogenous tissue repair machinery. Indeed, unless growth factors or drugs are added to their formulation, this class of biomaterials supports new tissue formation on the simple basis of the ability of their surface to act as a substrate for cell adhesion and proliferation. However, as mentioned before, this feature may not be sufficient to repair tissue when the biochemical signaling of cell cross-talk is impaired either by the extent of the damage (e.g. critical size defects of bony tissues) or by the pathological condition (e.g. diabetes). In addition, no biodegradable biomaterial has been designed to tune its rate of degradation to that of tissue ingrowth, which inevitably varies from patient to patient.

More recently, the simultaneous emergence of cell-based therapies (i.e. stem cells) and better understanding of the biological processes underlying tissue repair (i.e. growth factor signaling pathways) have triggered research towards tissue engineering constructs that are able to both jump-start tissue repair and lead to its completion with no need for permanent implants [6, 7].

2.2
Tissue Engineering

Tissue engineering has been defined as "a therapeutic application, where the tissue is either grown in a patient or outside the patient and transplanted" (Pittsburgh Tissue Engineering definition [8]). The main components of a tissue engineering construct have been identified by the Pittsburgh Tissue Engineering Initiative and by the American National Institute of Health [8] and clearly reflect the ambition to mimic the different components and functions of the original healthy tissue:

- biomaterials are used as substrates/scaffolds to promote cell adhesion, proliferation and differentiation, often mimicking the original histological properties of the extracellular matrix (ECM)
- cells (autologous cells or allogeneic cells) are the machinery producing new tissue upon biomaterial degradation
- biomolecules such as growth factors, drugs and genes are included to stimulate and regulate the activity of the cells entrapped in the biomaterial scaffold.
- engineering methods have to be implemented to assemble these components in a manner that satisfies the requirements for the tissue repair process and that can facilitate the storage and shipping of the construct from the manufacturing site to the surgical theatre.

These main components are also important in those cases where tissue formation is not meant to be achieved *in vivo*, but rather in a bioreactor system [9]. As the growth of tissues in bioreactor systems presents a series of challenges and cannot be dissociated from relatively invasive surgical implantation procedures, scientists are abandoning this concept and are focusing instead on injectable tissue engineering constructs that rely on minimally invasive surgical procedures and *in situ* tissue repair. For these reasons, tissue engineering approaches using bioreactor systems will not be considered in this chapter. The chapter will rather offer an overview of the technological approaches used for developing tissue engineering constructs, and will frame their application in the context of regeneration of tissues that are relevant to hand surgery.

2.3
Scaffold Fabrication Techniques

To fulfil its main role as a cell carrier during the implantation procedure and as a temporary cell support during the early phases of implantation, a biomaterial has to be able to mimic the ECM. This mimicry has to include the ECM architectural features and, ideally, its biochemical properties [10]. For example, in the case of biomaterials mimicking cancellous bone, their dominant feature is a macroporous 3D structure made of calcium phosphate-based materials such as hydroxyapatite [11]. Here, the macroporous structure mimics the trabecular architecture of cancellous bone, while the mineral phase presents the bone cells with their natural substrate. Conversely, in those cases where soft tissue needs to be repaired, biodegradable polymeric materials of natural and synthetic sources have been engineered. The use of biopolymers that are of either protein (e.g. collagen) or polysaccharide origin (e.g. hyaluronan) allows the exposure of bioligands with a role in cell adhesion, migration, proliferation and differentiation (see Section 2.5) [10–18].

In both cases, the typical engineering methods that have been employed to achieve 3D porous scaffolds are [7, 19]:

- fiber bonding: this is a technique where polymeric fibres are assembled by generating crosspoints with a second polymer. However, this method does not offer much control over the scaffold porosity
- emulsion freeze drying: this is a procedure where an emulsion dispersed in an aqueous phase is freeze dried to remove the water content and lead to the formation of a polymeric structure with interconnected pores up to 200 μm in size
- solvent casting/particulate leaching: this is accepted as one of the most suitable methods to produce scaffolds. In this procedure, a polymer solution in organic solvent is mixed with salt granules which are subsequently leached by dissolution to leave a degree of porosity up to 90%. The main limitation of this method is the efficiency of leaching of salt particles in relatively thick scaffolds
- high-pressure processing (also known as supercritical fluid technology): polymeric scaffolds can be prepared by this technique by applying a gas such as supercritical carbon dioxide to the dry polymer to form a single-phase polymer/gas solution. When the pressure is released, expansion of the dissolved carbon dioxide leads to formation of gas bubbles that generate uniform but poorly interconnected porosity within the polymeric matrix
- gas foaming/particulate leaching: this is a method where pores are formed by effervescent salt particles during their dissolution. Interconnected pores of a diameter ranging from 100 to 200 μm can usually be obtained by this technique
- thermally induced phase separation: this technique induces a thermodynamic demixing of a homogeneous polymer–solvent solution leading to the formation of two phases with different polymer concentrations. Demixing is obtained either by cooling below the solubility curve or by addition of an immiscible solvent. This technique, although recently improved by a coarsening step, does not lead to the

formation of large pores (maximum diameter 100 µm)

- electrospinning: this is a technique where a polymer solution or a molten polymer is drawn from a nozzle by gravity or mechanical pressure and in combination with an electric field, to form non-woven nanofiber matrices. During the process, the electric charge overcomes the surface tension of the polymer solution, transforming the polymer solution droplet into a polymer jet forming solid nanofibers upon solvent evaporation. Scaffolds with an interconnected porosity can be obtained with this method
- rapid prototyping: this process has been developed through computer-driven equipment which is able to construct 3D scaffolds by depositing droplets of molten material [19].

Other different approaches, applications and biological performances of scaffolds can be found in the literature [12, 20].

All these types of techniques share two main limitations:

- they are designed to achieve macroporosity favoring tissue ingrowth, but are not able to encapsulate cells into a single-cell 3D environment. In other words, cells seeded in macroporous scaffolds adhere to the pore wall, but still have part of their surface not in contact with elements of the ECM-mimicking environment. Therefore, as far as a single cell is concerned, these pores are still 2D environments and the cell morphology and activity may lose its natural features until it establishes either cell–ECM component contacts or cell-to-cell contacts
- they usually produce a porosity that is lost upon injection. Therefore, biomaterials engineered by these methods cannot be easily used as injectable formulations.

2.4
Cell Types in Tissue Engineering Constructs

The cells that are seeded into a biomaterial scaffold are a key component in a tissue engineering construct as they are the machinery responsible for jump-starting tissue repair. Biomaterial scaffolds for tissue engineering can be seeded with either differentiated or undifferentiated stem cells [21]. The choice of the cell type is dictated by the specific tissue needs. Thus far, no study on tissue engineering constructs has unequivocally provided indications about the advantages of using either differentiated or undifferentiated cells, and the benefit of using a cellularized scaffold is itself unclear. Indeed, cell therapy has been shown to only improve the clinical outcome in pathological conditions such as myocardial infarction and diseases of the nervous system where stem cell suspensions (with no biomaterial scaffold) have been injected [22, 23]. The use of autologous differentiated cells is linked to the ability to harvest sufficient amounts and to grow them *in vitro* for the purpose of generating the number required by the tissue engineering construct. However, the ability to proliferate these cells while maintaining a differentiated phenotype and their tissue regeneration potential is limited. For these reasons, most of the studies devoted to developing tissue engineering constructs have focused on the use of pluripotent or multipotent stem cells.

2.4.1
Embryonic Stem Cells

Following egg fertilization by a spermatozoon through an *in vitro* fertilization procedure (IVF), an embryo containing embryonic stem cells (ESCs) develops (Fig. 2.1a) [24]. Unlike cells that have already committed themselves to a specific phenotype, ESCs have a pluripotent (or totipotent) character that means they are able to differentiate into any type of cell phenotype and, therefore, have the potential to generate any type of tissue (Fig. 2.1a). Despite their enormous therapeutic potential, the use of these cells still presents limitations.

2.4.1.1
Technical Limitations

The method of culturing these cells is complicated by the need for a layer of feeder cells. These are usually murine fibroblasts. The contact between the underlying layer of feeder cells and the ESC is prone to the risk of cell fusion and transfer of genetic material from the cell of animal source to the human ESC (hESC). Furthermore, it is now widely accepted that preserving and controlling the undifferentiated hESC phenotype (namely cells positive to the markers: Nanog, Oct3/4, SOX2, SSEA1, Tra-1-68, Tra-1-81) in culture is a very difficult objective that limits the expansion of these cells in culture to reach the quantities necessary for most therapeutic interventions.

2.4.1.2
Ethical Concerns

The use of hESCs depends on the availability of unused embryos derived from IVF procedures. This is considered unacceptable by several groups in society because of their ethical and religious views.

2.4.1.3
Regulatory Issues

Because of both the technical limitations and ethical concerns, a strict regulatory framework is currently in place and constantly undergoing amendments. Such a regulatory framework will need to ensure a safe and ethical use of hESCs. Furthermore, growth media in which animal sera are used will need to be replaced by completely artificial media where the risk of transmissible disease is avoided.

2.4.2
Adult Mesenchymal Stem Cells

Adult mesenchymal stem cells (MSCs) are progenitor cells that are still able to differentiate into different cell phenotypes and to participate in tissue regeneration (Fig. 2.1b) [25]. Unlike ESCs, MSC potency is considered to be of a multipotent character rather than pluripotent. This means that MSCs are already committed towards specific cell phenotypes and, therefore, their ability to regenerate tissue is limited to those specific cell types (Fig. 2.1b). Although most of the tissues have a stem cell niche that is activated upon tissue damage, the main source of stem cells for therapeutic use is the bone marrow. As for ESCs, MSCs have specific markers of expression such as, for example, STRO-1. However, their marker profile is still not complete and more information is required to define a "true" MSC. A profile has been quite exhaustively obtained for a particular lineage of progenitor cells present in the bone marrow; that

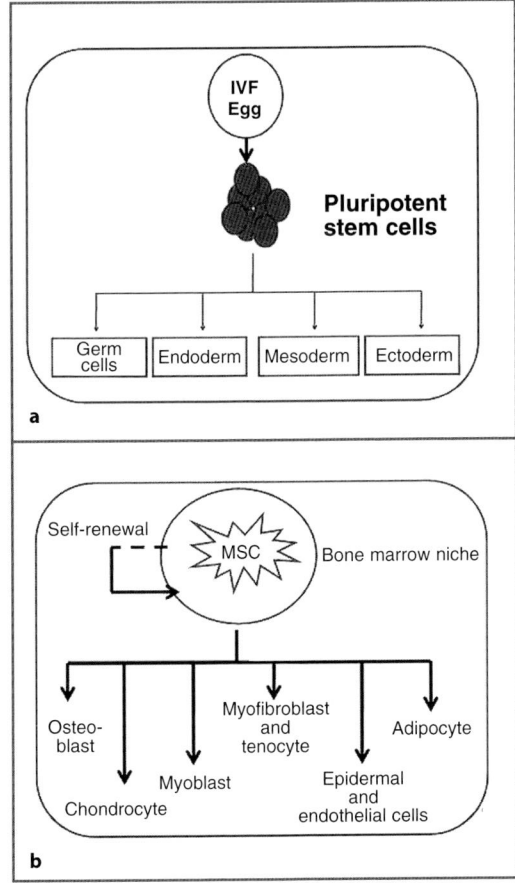

Fig. 2.1 Source and differentiation trees of embryonic stem cells (**a**) and adult hematopoietic and mesenchymal stromal stem cells (MSCs) (**b**)

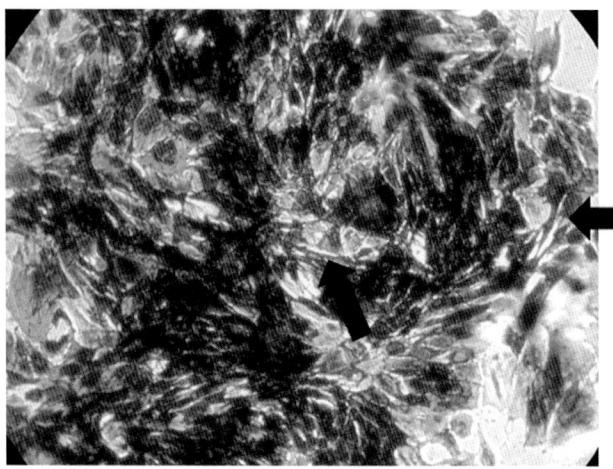

Fig. 2.2 Typical morphology of adult MSCs isolated from human bone marrow. *Arrows* indicate a typical spindle-like cell indicating culture contamination by myofibroblasts. Micrograph kindly provided by Mr. Matthew Ilsley

is the hemapoietic stem cells (HSCs) which express CD133 and CD34 as markers [26]. These cells play a fundamental role in angiogenesis, a process that is important in sustaining the repair of tissues relevant to hand surgery, such as bone, nerves and skin [27]. These cells are available in a quiescent state, but they are mobilized from their niche to proliferate and differentiate into endothelial cells in several cell lineages of the immune system, as well as into red blood cells.

The therapeutic use of MSCs still presents some limitations which, as for the hESCs, are mainly linked to the need for their expansion *in vitro* in an undifferentiated state. Currently, a significant percentage of cultured MSCs tend to differentiate into (or are contaminated by) fibroblasts, thus limiting their use for obtaining other cell types (Fig. 2.2). Future understanding of the culturing requirements for controlling the MSC phenotype *in vitro* will be the key to the use of these cells in clinics.

2.4.3
Induced Pluripotent Stem Cells

More recently, alongside the use of hESCs and MSCs, so-called induced pluripotent stem cells (iPSCs) have been proposed for therapeutic applications [28]. These cells are human somatic cells (fibroblasts) where the pluripotency is retrieved by virus-mediated transcription of some of the genes conferring pluripotency to the ESC (i.e. *SOX2* and *OCT3/4* genes). Although iPSCs may resolve ethical controversies, they still raise technical and regulatory issues. From a technical viewpoint, the rate of transfection of the genes may not necessarily be satisfactory, while the risks associated with the use of viral vectors may make regulatory approval difficult to achieve. Furthermore, there would inevitably be additional costs in the commercialization phase of these engineered cells, as a result of the requirements of the transfection procedure.

More information about the biological characteristics and therapeutic potential of hESCs, MSCs and iPSCs can be found in comprehensive review papers [25–28].

2.5
Biomimetic Materials, Bioligands and Bioactive Molecules for Tissue Engineering Constructs

In an attempt to reproduce the natural environment hosting tissue regeneration and repair, 3D macroporous scaffolds of polymeric (natural and synthetic origin) and ceramic materials have been engineered (see Section 2.3). Despite improvement of their features, these scaffolds do not mimic the complex composition of bioligands and growth factors that cells are exposed to during tissue formation. In particular, the scaffolds do not offer the correct presentation of bioligands that are able to regulate cell adhesion and migration; they also lack the soluble biochemical stimuli that control tissue repair.

In this section, an overview of some of the most important polymeric and ceramic biomaterials is presented, together with some alternative synthetic peptides that are able to mimic the bioligands present in biopolymers. These synthetic bioligands can be used as functionalization molecules for biomaterial surfaces. Furthermore, the important role of growth factors and other bioactive molecules of natural and synthetic origin in the tissue engineering construct will also be discussed.

2.5.1
Collagen

Collagen is the main component of the ECM of most soft and hard connective tissues [29]. Although there are many types of collagens, collagen type I has been the type considered for most technological applications in tissue engineering. The ability of collagen to act as a substrate for cell adhesion and mineralization during bone formation depends on the presence of specific functional groups in this protein. Specific amino acid sequences act as bioligands for cell receptors (i.e. cell membrane integrins), while other functionalities or collagen-bound non-collagenous proteins work as nucleation points for the formation of hydroxyapatite crystals. For these reasons, 3D collagen scaffolds have been engineered either as monolithic materials or in combination with other macromolecular components of the ECM, and used to seed cells for the engineering of both soft and hard tissues.

In its natural conformation, this protein is characterized by a repetitive amino acid sequence in which hydroxyproline ensures the folding of fibrils into a triple helix. Collagen fibrils are then assembled into fibers, bundles, fascicles and mesh, thus playing a role as scaffold for cells.

However, collagens also play an important role in regulating cell activity and, as a consequence, tissue repair. For example, type I collagen has been shown to promote angiogenesis both *in vitro* and *in vivo* [30]. This angiogenic potential has been ascribed to the ability of this protein to control endothelial cell behavior by promoting ligation and, possibly, clustering of the cells. It is known that this control is exerted through binding of plasmalemma $\alpha_1\beta_1/\alpha_2\beta_1$ integrin receptors to the amino acid sequence -GFPGER- of the collagen fibril.

Furthermore, it has been suggested that type I collagen may also contribute to cell functions by molecular mechanotransduction [31]. Recent evidence shows that these stimuli regulate the cytoskeleton and, as a consequence, the expression of particular genes within the cell nucleus. The most well-known amino acid sequence present in type I collagen, as well as in other ECM proteins such as fibronectin, is the -RGD-sequence. This triplet ensures relatively strong cell adhesion to the ECM as a consequence of its recognition by the plasmalemma integrins.

Type II collagen is one of the main components of the pericellular matrix (PCM) surrounding chondrocytes in articular cartilage, a tissue layer that is believed to have fine control in the chondrocyte differentiated phenotype [32]. To mimic the chondron (the histological unit in which chondrocytes are naturally located), fabricated microspheres of collagen have been used as carriers for hMSC microencapsulation [33]. The collagen microspheres have been shown to induce hMSC pre-differentiation into a chondrocyte-like phenotype *in vitro*. Other approaches towards cartilage regeneration have been pursued, where hMSCs were encapsulated in type II collagen fibers [34].

Type IV collagen is mainly found in the basement membranes of epithelium and endothelium, where it forms supramolecular networks able to control cell adhesion, migration and differentiation [35, 36]. Like the other types of collagen, type IV collagen forms complexes with other macromolecules to offer structural support to the tissue and to regulate cell functions.

2.5.2
Fibrin

Fibrin is the main component of the blood clot and is formed through enzyme-driven activation, polymerization and crosslinking of fibrinogen [37].

Once the fibrin mesh is formed, platelets are entrapped to stop the bleeding. Fibrin is also able to bind biochemicals, such as growth factors, that are important for tissue repair and, therefore, is able to produce chemotactic gradients for recruitment of stem cells as well as stimulation of tissue cell migration and differentiation [38]. For these reasons, autologous clots and commercially available fibrin glue have been used in many surgical applications. These biological properties, together with the relatively elastic character of the fibrin mesh, have also prompted the use of fibrin-based biomaterials as scaffolds for tissue engineering in soft and hard tissue applications [39].

2.5.3
Glycosaminoglycans (GAGs) and Proteoglycans (PGNs)

GAGs and PGNs participate in many biological processes including wound healing. As in the case of fibrin, GAGs and PGNs are also able to bind growth factors and, consequently, to control cell activity [40]. In addition, GAGs regulate cell–ECM interactions and activation of chemokines, enzymes and growth factors [41].

GAGs, and to some extent PGNs, have a relatively high hydrophilic nature that makes them able to retain water within tissues, particularly in articular cartilage, thus contributing to their biomechanical properties.

Among the GAGs most used in tissue engineering it is worth mentioning hyaluronan (HA). HA is a relatively high molecular weight glycosaminoglycan composed of repeating monomeric units of D-glucuronic acid, β1–3 and N-acetyl-D-glucosamine β1–4 [42]. HA plays a key role in tissue development, homeostasis and repair. For example, through its specific interactions with CD44 cell receptors, HA is able to promote cell recruitment. High molecular weight HA ($>2 \times 10^6$ Daltons) favors the activation of endothelial cells and, therefore, angiogenesis [41, 43].

For these reasons, HA has been used in regenerative medicine to induce tissue repair [44].

2.5.4
Ceramics

Ceramic materials have been widely used to fabricate macroporous scaffolds for bone tissue engineering [11, 20]. The rationale underpinning the use of these biomaterials is their chemical nature, which is very similar to that of bone mineralized matrix. Therefore, the use of these materials can be regarded as another strategy to provide the cells with an environment similar to that of the original tissue to be repaired. The most common ceramic biomaterials used for bone tissue engineering are calcium phosphate-based biomaterials and bioactive glasses [11, 20, 45]. Both these classes have been shown to stimulate bone formation by providing either a suitable substrate for the cells (calcium-phosphate osteoconductivity) or a stimulation of their activity (bioglass osteogenic potential). Due to their ability to partially fulfil the required mechanical properties, the most frequently used ceramics for tissue engineering are hydroxyapatite and beta-tricalcium phosphate as well as scaffolds obtained by combination of these two materials. However, due to their brittle character, ceramic scaffolds are not satisfactory in load-bearing applications and their implantation requires relatively invasive surgery. Recently, some studies have been performed to optimize injectable calcium phosphate cements that can be implanted by a minimally invasive procedure. However, these calcium phosphate cements set *in vivo*, and the setting reaction is incompatible with cell survival. Therefore, these cements cannot be used as carriers for cell delivery.

Nevertheless, a recent seven-year follow-up clinical study has shown good performance of bone tissue engineering constructs where 3D ceramic scaffolds were seeded with hMSCs for the purpose of facilitating tissue repair in severe damage of long bones [46]. Such a study may be considered an interesting proof of concept for critical-size bone defect repair in hand surgery where the surgical procedure is, *per se*, invasive.

2.5.5
Synthetic Bioligands

Although natural polymers have biological properties making them suitable for tissue engineering constructs, their use is impaired by several drawbacks. First, batch-to-batch variations can reduce the reproducibility of their clinical performance. Secondly, the inevitable extraction and engineering processes that they undergo in order to be made available as biomaterials may negatively alter their physicochemical properties and, as a consequence, lead to a partial or complete loss of their biocompatibility. Thirdly, when extracted from natural sources, they may become vehicles for transmissible diseases. Finally, regardless of their animal or recombinant source, they can be obtained only after laborious and relatively expensive processing. These drawbacks significantly limit their use in the manufacturing of tissue engineering constructs where the tuning of cell activity is dependent on a finely tuned balance of biochemical events. For these reasons, several research groups worldwide have tried to functionalize the surface of synthetic materials with specific peptide sequences able to mimic the bioligand activity that is at the root of most of the natural polymer biological properties [47–49]. This approach is intended to bring together the advantages of using relatively cheap and highly reproducible synthetic materials with the presence of biospecific cues able to regulate cell activity.

For example, poly(ethylene glycol) (PEG) hydrogels have been functionalized by a combination of integrin-binding sites to ensure cell adhesion (i.e. -RGDSP- peptide). Later, other properties of the ECM such as those of binding important growth factors and responding to cell activity were mimicked. PEG-bis-vinylsulfone has been crosslinked with a peptide containing three cysteine residues [17], making the scaffold susceptible to cleavage by cell-associated plasmin, a protease that is able to digest ECM protein components. As a consequence, cells contacting this type of hydrogel were able to invade its network, where they interact with grafted adhesion peptides which were linked to the main polymer backbone through plasmin-resistant peptides. The bone repair potential of these hydrogels has been improved by their functionalization with heparin, which is able to bind a potent bone growth factor, bone morphogenetic protein-2 (BMP-2) [17].

The amino acid sequence -RGD-, which is present in collagen and other ECM proteins, has also been grafted onto 3D alginate gels to favor bone ingrowth through both a higher cell adhesion and activation of relevant genes [47]. A review in the literature [48] offers a very comprehensive overview of the different grafting methods, and highlights the importance of the degree of exposure of -RGD- peptides to cells. In addition to the -RGD- sequence, other amino acid sequences have been shown to promote cell interaction with surfaces. In particular, biospecific interactions of osteoblasts have been obtained by the use of either the -FHRRIKA- sequence, which promotes osteoblast migration rather than adhesion [50], or the -KRSR- sequence, which promotes osteoblast adhesion. FHRRIKA and KRSR have in common an ability to bind proteoglycans [11, 50].

To improve MSC spreading, -KRSR- and -FHRRIKA- peptides were combined with -RGD- onto hydroxyapatite surfaces, but the combination of these peptides did not achieve any enhanced spreading of MSCs. Osteoblast adhesion assays on acellular bone matrix using a novel peptide carrying the X-B-B-B-X-B-B-X motif (where B is a basic amino acid and X is a non-basic residue) were shown to promote proteoglycan-mediated osteoblast adhesion more efficiently than the -KRSR- sequence, which is considered to be a heparan sulfate-binding peptide [49].

These studies demonstrate that the functionalization of tissue engineering constructs by these functionalization peptides may not be desirable, and careful studies need to be performed depending on the targeted tissue repair. Furthermore, the synthesis and storage of these relatively unstable peptides may limit their clinical use.

2.5.6
Bioactive Molecules

Mimicry of the ECM has not been limited to the structure of bioligand-exposing macromolecules. Proteins playing a key role in the biomineralization process have also been mimicked in the structure of biomaterials for bone applications. Interpenetrating nanostructured architecture, using relatively simple anionic polypeptides that mimic the polyanionic character of most of the calcium-binding proteins have been used [51].

Since its infancy, the field of tissue engineering and its relative technological approaches have been dependent on the ability to control the behavior of the progenitor and differentiated cells upon their seeding throughout the 3D scaffold. It was soon recognized that fine control can be obtained only through exploitation of the biochemical signaling that characterizes the repair process in all tissues. For this purpose, tissue engineering constructs have been complemented by the introduction of either relevant growth factors or their synthetic analogues. Growth factors of natural or recombinant origin have been used in an attempt to stimulate cell proliferation and differentiation. Among these, it is worth mentioning transforming growth factor (TGF)-beta 1 and BMP-2 for bone regeneration, vascular endothelial growth factor (VEGF) for angiogenesis, insulin-like growth factor (IGF)-1 for cartilage repair, basic fibroblast growth factor (FGF) for skin regeneration, and nerve growth factor (NGF) for peripheral nerve repair. However, due to their relatively unstable nature, the risk of transmissible diseases and/or their relatively high costs, these growth factors may be difficult to use in the large-scale production of tissue engineering constructs. For these reasons, more recently, peptide sequences that are able to act as analogues of specific growth factors have been proposed [52] (Table 2.1).

To be effective, both growth factors and their analogues need to become rapidly available to the cells and sustain their bioactivity over a relatively long period of time. For these reasons, several strategies have been adopted to ensure a protracted release of these bioactive molecules. Molecular encapsulation and reversible conjugation are the most frequently used approaches. However, due to the relatively low molecular weight of these peptides, encapsulation may not be able to control their release, especially in macroporous 3D scaffolds. In an attempt to improve the delivery kinetics upon encapsulation, functional groups able to reversibly bind growth factors (e.g. heparin) have been added to the polymeric scaffold surface. Also, the transfection of cells with

Table 2.1 Peptide analogues of growth factors

Peptide sequence/name	Function
-GGSKPPGTSS-CONH$_2$	Bone marrow homing/cell differentiation
-GGPPSSTKT-CONH$_2$	Bone marrow homing/cell differentiation
QPWLEQAYYSTF	Stimulates endothelial cell proliferation/angiogenesis
KLTWQELYQLKYKGI	VEGF analogue/angiogenesis
SSSR	IGF-1 mimicking/corneal epithelial cell proliferation
NSVNSKIPKACCVPTELSAI	BMP-2 analogue/osteogenesis
CTCE-0214	SDF-1 peptide analogue/survival of cord blood hemoprogenitor cells

genes for specific growth factors has been considered. This approach would ensure that, once seeded within the scaffold mesh, cells like the osteoblasts could ensure the secretion of higher levels of growth factors such as VEGF, which is one of the key factors for angiogenesis. However, because of the manipulation of their genome, there may be safety issues associated with this strategy [53].

Finally, the important role of drugs cannot be ignored. Over the years, pharmaceutical compounds able to direct cell activity have been explored and have reached clinical practice, improving and saving the lives of many patients worldwide. Indeed, attempts have been made to use some pharmaceutically active substances and plant molecules as functionalization molecules of biomaterials. Their role may become fundamental in the development of future tissue engineering constructs.

2.6
Conclusions

Extensive research activity is currently in progress worldwide to develop tissue engineering constructs for the repair of both soft and hard tissues. The combination of expertise in multidisciplinary environments will be a key factor in the development of clinical products. Biomaterials with tuned physicochemical properties will need to be made available to provide efficient encapsulation systems for cells. The use of bioactive molecules, either grafted to the scaffold or released from it in a controlled manner, seems also to be necessary to control repair of the damaged tissues. Regulatory and ethical issues will also need to be dealt with to ensure that the development of these products will be carried out with full respect of the patient's needs and rights. In the specific case of hand surgery, careful consideration will be required to define those cases where tissue engineering products can lead to a significant improvement in the patient's recovery. Case-by-case assessment of the patient's clinical conditions, surgical requirement (e.g. ease of handling of the product) and overall costs of the products will need to be considered by both medical companies and clinicians.

References

1. Murray PM (2003) New-generation implant arthroplasties for the finger joints. J Am Acad Orthop Surg 11:295–301.
2. Mishra V, Kuiper JH, Kelly CP (2003) Influence of core suture material and peripheral repair technique on the strength of Kessler flexor tendon repair. J Hand Surg 28:357–362.
3. Bertleff MJOE, Meek MF, Nicolai JPA (2005) A prospective clinical evaluation of biodegradable neurolac nerve guides for sensory nerve repair in the hand. J Hand Surg 30:513–518.
4. Conolly WB, Rath S (1991) Silastic implant arthroplasty for post-traumatic stiffness of the finger joints. J Hand Surg 16:286–292.
5. Hubbell JA (1998) Synthetic biodegradable polymers for tissue engineering and drug delivery. Curr Opin Solid State Mater Sci 3(3):246–251.
6. Langer R, Vacanti JP (1993) Tissue engineering. Science 260:920–926.
7. Chung HJ, Park TG (2007) Surface engineered and drug releasing pre-fabricated scaffolds for tissue engineering. Adv Drug Del Res 59:249–262.
8. Pittsburgh Tissue Engineering Institute. www.ptei.org (accessed 15 June 2009).
9. Hutmacher DW, Singh H (2008) Computational fluid dynamics for improved bioreactor design and 3D culture. Trends Biotechnol 26:166–172.
10. Sawyer AA, Hennessy KM, Bellis SL (2007) The effect of adsorbed serum proteins, RGD and proteoglycan-binding peptides on the adhesion of mesenchymal stem cells to hydroxyapatite. Biomaterials 28:383–392.
11. Ehrbar M, Lutolf MP, Rizzi SC et al (2008) Artificial extracellular matrices for bone tissue engineering. Bone 42:S72.
12. Lee J, Cuddihy MJ, Kotov NA (2008) Three-dimensional cell culture matrices: State of the art. Tissue Eng Part B Rev 14:61–86.
13. Lutolf MP, Hubbell JA (2005) Synthetic biomaterials as instructive extracellular microenvironments for morphogenesis in tissue engineering. Nature Biotechnol 23:47–55.
14. Hubbell JA (2003) Materials as morphogenetic guides in tissue engineering. Curr Opin Biotechnol 14:551–558.
15. Lutolf MR, Weber FE, Schmoekel HG et al (2003) Repair of bone defects using synthetic mimetics of collagenous extracellular matrices. Nature Biotechnol 21:513–518.
16. Lutolf MP, Lauer-Fields JL, Schmoekel HG et al (2003) Synthetic matrix metalloproteinase-sensitive hydrogels for the conduction of tissue regeneration: engineering cell-invasion characteristics. Proc Natl Acad Sci U S A 100:5413–5418.
17. Pratt AB, Weber FE, Schmoekel HG et al (2004) Synthetic extracellular matrices for in situ tissue engineering. Biotechnol Bioeng 86:27–36.
18. Rizzi SC, Ehrbar M, Halstenberg S et al (2006) Recombinant protein-co-PEG networks as cell-adhesive and proteolytically degradable hydrogel matrixes. Part II: Biofunctional characteristics. Biomacromolecules 7:3019–3029.
19. Chua CK, Sudarmadji N, Leong KF (2008) Functionally graded scaffolds: the challenges in design and fabrication processes. In: Bártolo PJ, Mateus AJ, Batista FDC et al (eds) Virtual and rapid manufacturing: advanced research in virtual and rapid prototyping. Monographs in engineering, water and earth sciences. Taylor and Francis, London, pp115–120.
20. Jones JR, Gentleman E, Polak J (2007) Bioactive glass scaffolds for bone regeneration. Elements 3:393–399.
21. Kochar PG (2004) What are stem cells? www.csa.com/discoveryguides/stemcell/overview.php (accessed 29 May 2009).
22. Forrester JS, Price MJ, Makkar RR (2003) Stem cell repair of infarcted myocardium: an overview for clinicians. Circulation 108:1139–1145.
23. Lindvall O, Kokaia Z (2006) Stem cells for the treatment of neurological disorders. Nature 441:1094–1096.

24. Gerecht-Nir S, Itskoviz-Eldor J (2004) Cell therapy using human embryonic stem cells. Transpl Immunol 12:203–209.
25. Ratajczak MZ, Zuba-Surma EK, Wysoczynski M et al (2008) Hunt for pluripotent stem cell – regenerative medicine search for almighty cell. J Autoimmunol 30:151–162.
26. Hines M, Nielsen L, Cooper-White J (2008) The hematopoietic stem cell niche: what are we trying to replicate? J Chem Technol Biotechnol 83:421–443.
27. Kim S, Von Recum H (2007) Endothelial stem cells and precursors for tissue engineering: cell source, differentiation, selection, and application. Tissue Eng Part B Rev 14:133–147.
28. Yu J, Vodyanik MA, Smuga-Otto K et al (2007) Induced pluripotent stem cells derived from somatic cells. Science 318:1917–1920.
29. Benjamin M, Kaiser E, Milz S (2008) Structure–function relationships in tendons: a review. J Anat 212:211–228.
30. Twardowski T, Fertala A, Orgel JPRO, Antonio JDS (2007) Type I collagen and collagen mimetics as angiogenesis promoting superpolymers. Curr Pharm Design 13:3608–3621.
31. Peyton SR, Ghajar CM, Khatiwala CB, Putnam AJ (2007) The emergence of ECM mechanics and cytoskeletal tension as important regulators of cell function. Cell Biochem Biophys 47:300–320.
32. Guilak F, Alexopoulos LG, Upton ML et al (2006) The pericellular matrix as a transducer of biomechanical and biochemical signals in articular cartilage. Ann NY Acad Sci 1068:498–512.
33. Hui TY, Cheung KMC, Cheung WL et al (2008) In vitro chondrogenic differentiation of human mesenchymal stem cells in collagen microspheres: Influence of cell seeding density and collagen concentration. Biomaterials 29:3201–3212.
34. Chang CF, Lee MW, Kuo PY et al (2007) Three-dimensional collagen fiber remodeling by mesenchymal stem cells requires the integrin–matrix interaction. J Biomed Mater Res A 80A:466–474.
35. Khoshnoodi J, Pedchenko V, Hudson BG (2008) Mammalian collagen IV. Microsc Res Tech 71:357–370.
36. LeBleu VS, MacDonald B, Kalluri R (2007) Structure and function of basement membranes. Exp Biol Med 232:1121–1127.
37. Lim BBC, Lee EH, Sotomayor M, Schulten K (2008) Molecular basis of fibrin clot elasticity. Structure 16:449–459.
38. Nurden AT, Nurden P, Sanchez M et al (2008) Platelets and wound healing. Front Biosci 13:3532–3548.
39. Zhao HG, Ma L, Zhou J et al (2008) Fabrication and physical and biological properties of fibrin gel derived from human plasma. Biomed Mat 3:15001.
40. Yung S, Chan TM (2007) Glycosaminoglycans and proteoglycans: overlooked entities? Perit Dial Int 27(Suppl 2):S104–109.
41. Taylor KR, Gallo RL (2006) Glycosaminoglycans and their proteoglycans: host-associated molecular patterns for initiation and modulation of inflammation. FASEB J 20:9–22.
42. Bastow ER, Byers S, Golub SB et al (2008) Hyaluronan synthesis and degradation in cartilage and bone. Cell Mol Life Sci 65:395–413.
43. Slevin M, Krupinski J, Gaffney J et al (2007) Hyaluronan-mediated angiogenesis in vascular disease: uncovering RHAMM and CD44 receptor signaling pathways. Matrix Biol 26:58–68.
44. Jiang D, Liang J, Noble PW (2007) Hyaluronan in tissue injury and repair. Annu Rev Cell Dev Biol 23:435–461.
45. Teixeira S, Oliveira S, Ferraz MP, Monteiro FJ (2008) Three dimensional macroporous calcium phosphate scaffolds for bone tissue engineering. In: Daculsi G, Layrolle P (eds) Bioceramics 20, Parts 1 and 2. Book series: key engineering materials, pp947–950. Trans Tech Publications Inc, Zurich.
46. Quarto R, Mastrogiacomo M, Cancedda R et al (2001) Repair of large bone defects with the use of autologous bone marrow stromal cells. N Engl J Med 344:385–386.

47. Evangelista MB, Hsiong SX, Fernandes R et al (2007) Upregulation of bone cell differentia-
     tion through immobilization within a synthetic extracellular matrix. Biomaterials 28:3644–3655.
48. Hersel U, Dahmen C, Kessler H (2003) RGD modified polymers: biomaterials for stimulat-
     ed cell adhesion and beyond. Biomaterials 24:4385–4415.
49. Dettin M, Conconi MT, Gambaretto R et al (2002) Novel osteoblast-adhesive peptides for den-
     tal/orthopedic biomaterials. J Biomed Mater Res 60:466–471.
50. Rezania A, Healy KE (1999) Biomimetic peptide surfaces that regulate adhesion, spreading,
     cytoskeletal organization, and mineralization of the matrix deposited by osteoblast-like cells.
     Biotechnol Prog 15:19–32.
51. Pollock JF, Healy KE (2009) Biomimetic and bio-responsive materials in regenerative med-
     icine. In: Santin M (ed) Strategies in regenerative medicine. Integrating biology with materi-
     als science. Springer, Milan, pp97–154.
52. Lloyd AW, Oliver GWJ, Standen G et al (2008) Biomaterial with functionalised surfaces.
     WO/2008/068531. World Intellectual Property Organization, www.wipo.int/pctdb/en/wo.jsp?
     WO=2008068531 (accessed 13 June 2009).
53. Matsumoto R, Omura T, Yoshiyama M et al (2005) Vascular endothelial growth factor–express-
     ing mesenchymal stem cell transplantation for the treatment of acute myocardial infarction.
     Arterioscl Thromb Vasc Biol 25:1168–1173.

The Finite Element Method for the Design of Biomedical Devices

3

F. Mollica and L. Ambrosio

Abstract Some of the design techniques available today are suitable for application in the biomedical field. Among these, the most interesting ones make use of the computer for drawing, simulating, and manufacturing, and are commonly called computer-aided engineering, or CAE. The finite element method (FEM) is often at the heart of these powerful methods and is treated in detail within this chapter.

The treatment of this subject in the present chapter will avoid the mathematical framework that constitutes the basis of FEM. The intention of the authors is to give a practical viewpoint on FEM; thus a sample problem will be used in order to describe both the sequence of operations needed in a FEM analysis and some of the fundamental issues that are involved. The sample problem has been chosen in a subject that is not too far from the interests of the readers. However, it must be pointed out that the treatment of this problem is functional only to the presentation of FEM; thus the problem is simplified in order to make FEM more clearly understandable, and consequently the results of the sample problem cannot be assumed to hold in a realistic setting.

Keywords Computer-aided Engineering • Design • Finite Element Method • Mesh • Numerical Methods • Refinement • Strain • Stress

3.1
Introduction

The steps involved in the path towards a novel biomedical device comprise, early in the process, close interaction between the medical doctor and the engineer. Typically, the medical doctor expresses the need for a certain device that can improve his work, and comes up with the basic idea for the device itself. The engineer can then help in the realization of the idea, by selecting the right materials and correct dimensions in order that the device can be developed and will perform as desired for a long duration and in an economically viable way. These tasks are in fact part of the process of design, which, at a very basic level, consists of choosing the shape of the device, together with its dimensions and material (or materials).

F. Mollica (✉)
Department of Engineering, University of Ferrara, Ferrara, Italy

A. Merolli, T.J. Joyce (eds), *Biomaterials in Hand Surgery.*
© Springer-Verlag Italia 2009

In order to carry out the design process correctly, many engineering fundamentals will have to be exploited, together with the designer's experience, and the whole procedure is quite complex. Significant support comes from computer-aided engineering, or CAE, i.e., the use of information technology in the form of suitable computer software (for drawing, analyzing, simulating, planning, etc) that helps the design engineer accomplish his tasks. Currently, CAE in the form of CAD (computer-aided design, used mainly for technical drawing) or CAM (computer-aided manufacturing) are widespread in the industry as well as in the scientific literature related to design.

An important part of CAE is stress analysis on components and assemblies. Stress, indicated by σ, is a measure of the internal forces that are generated within a certain body due to the forces that are applied externally and, in certain particular cases, can be thought of as the external force F divided by the area on which the force is acting, A:

$$\sigma = \frac{F}{A}$$

Being able to calculate the stress in a material is important for two reasons: firstly, if the stress is known one can calculate the deformations of the body, i.e., how the body moves under the effect of the external forces; secondly, all materials fail once a limiting value for the stress is reached, thus, knowing the stress, one can predict whether or not the component will break. Stress analysis in CAE is usually performed using the finite element method (FEM). This method allows simulation of the mechanical behavior of a certain part subject to external loads, once its geometrical features and material properties are known. As a consequence, the final result of FEM is not the final design but rather the verification that a certain design meets the requirements and specifications that have been set.

More generally speaking, the design of a new part almost always has as an intermediate point the development of one or more prototypes, i.e., models of the part that can be used solely for preliminary testing purposes: the prototypes must undergo extensive experimental testing to make sure that all the possible relevant faults are revealed and taken care of before commercialization. Despite prototyping being a very expensive step in the design process, in terms of the cost of the prototype itself and especially in terms of the time needed before final commercialization, it is absolutely necessary, particularly in settings where extensive risks are at stake, such as the biomedical field. The application of simulations through the FEM allows one to foresee the conditions that the component will undergo once in use, and can be thus seen as a very convenient way to reduce the number of costly prototypes, rendering the whole design process faster and more economic.

The current scientific literature in almost every branch of science and engineering is becoming increasingly involved with FEM. Biomedical disciplines are also employing this powerful method through interdisciplinary subjects that share common boundaries with technical areas, such as biomedical engineering or theoretical biology. Here, thanks to its specific properties, FEM is rapidly gaining the same success it obtained in the disciplines where it originated and was first applied, such as structural mechanics and heat transfer. Clearly, the most wide-ranging applications are in those areas where mechanical loading is a key parameter, for instance orthopedics and dentistry. Certainly, in addition to FEM's unique properties, much of the success in this field is due to the great number of commercial FEM packages that are available today. These have the great advantage of also making FEM available to personnel who are not trained specifically in the mathematical subtleties of the method. Nevertheless, it is clear that running meaningful and reliable FEM simulations should not be done without, at the very least, a basic knowledge of the method.

In this chapter we will mainly focus on the application of FEM to the design and simulation of biomedical devices. It is not the intention of the authors to provide an exhaustive knowledge of the method. The reader who is interested in gaining a deeper understanding is advised to check the books that are listed at the end of the chapter. This chapter is, rather, intended to give a taste of what FEM really is, and, more importantly, an introduction to what it can and cannot do.

3.2
What is the Finite Element Method?

Strictly speaking, the finite element method is a method to solve a certain group of mathematical equations that are called "differential equations", i.e., in general terms, equations in which the unknown or unknowns are functions that appear in the equations together with their derivatives. This is the first important issue: FEM limits itself to solving a certain number of equations. This means, for example, that if the equations are not the right ones, it cannot be expected that the FEM results are accurate. In other words, it is inappropriate to state that a particular problem, such as the deformation of a vascular prosthesis or the stresses and strains in a hip prosthesis, has been solved with FEM. FEM merely solves the differential equations that describe that particular problem. In fact, these are very often the real issue. So where do the equations come from? And why do we need them in the first place?

The laws of physics have been formulated in order to enable us to understand and thus predict and possibly control physical phenomena. The laws of gravitation, due to Newton, and electromagnetism, due to Maxwell, are examples of the laws of physics: a given phenomenon is explained in terms of a certain number of measurable quantities that are believed to be controlling it. The basis of the formulation of the laws of physics is the observation of nature, together with logical interpretations of the observed phenomena. Moreover, before being definitively accepted, every theory is put to the test with a series of experiments that can disprove it at any point in the process; therefore, once a theory is accepted it can be a very useful model of reality.

Nevertheless, in order for a theory to be effective, it must be cast in a form that allows its use. This is given by mathematics, usually through a suitable equation or system of equations that connect the variables of interest. The predictions on the physical phenomenon we are interested in come from solving these mathematical equations, which are normally called a "mathematical model". An easy example is Newton's laws of motion, in particular the well-known second law:

$$F = ma$$

where F is the net force acting on a point object, m is its mass, and a its acceleration. This equation tells us that when the force acting on an object of given mass is known, one can calculate its acceleration and hence its motion.

An important point about Newton's second law is its simplicity: acceleration can be calculated from force and mass through trivial calculations. Simplicity is extremely important: if a theory is so complex that it cannot be solved to obtain useful predictions, it would be appropriate to consider such a theory as completely useless. This is exactly why a good model should be made as simple as possible (but not any simpler), one of the scientific applications of Occam's razor[1].

Complications, unfortunately, do come into the picture, and in some fields are unavoidable. An example is in fact the biomedical field. Here phenomena are governed by a plethora of variables and it is really hard to distinguish the ones that are actually important from those that can be neglected as a first approximation. A source of complexity is also the mathematical setting. As a suitable example, let us consider the mathematical model arising in the theory of heat transfer, which describes the conduction of heat in a body:

$$\frac{\partial T}{\partial t} = \alpha \left(\frac{\partial T}{\partial x^2} + \frac{\partial T}{\partial y^2} + \frac{\partial T}{\partial z^2} \right)$$

This equation is commonly indicated as the heat equation: T is the main variable, i.e., temperature, t is time, α is the thermal diffusivity, and the triplet x, y, and z denotes the position within the body.

With this equation one assumes that temperature is a function that in general depends on time as well as the position within the body, $T = T(x,y,z,t)$. In order to formulate predictions, the heat equation must be solved for T at every point of the "domain", i.e., the body in which heat transfer is taking place, and for each instant of time. As the reader can imagine, this can become extremely difficult if it has to be done analytically, i.e., exactly, especially if the domain has a very complex shape. As an alternative, the solution can be sought using "numerical methods", i.e., methods that make use of the computer. These are, by their very nature, approximate methods. The FEM is simply one of these numerical methods, probably the most used and well known.

3.3
The Main Steps Involved in a FEM Analysis

In order to provide the reader with a practical knowledge of FEM, the main steps of a FEM analysis will be described in relation to a sample problem: the loading of a cemented hip prosthesis during standing up. We will look for the displacements in the

---

[1]   Occam was a 14th century English logician and Franciscan friar who stated that one should not increase beyond what is necessary the number of entitites required to explain anything.

hip prosthesis and for the stresses in the bone holding the prosthesis. This problem, though, merely serves as an example that will guide us through the application of FEM; this cannot be overemphasized. As a consequence we will simplify the problem considerably, to the point that the results we will obtain cannot be considered reliable from a clinical point of view. It is not the intention of the authors to provide the readers with an accurate representation of the stress fields arising in bone due to the presence of a prosthesis; there are plenty of excellent papers in the scientific literature that are interested in this. We just want to show, hopefully in a clear way, the procedure used to perform such an analysis.

The applied forces, for instance, will be approximated as a single point force applied on the head of the prosthesis along the vertical direction. Bone will also be considered as constituted only by compact bone, so we will neglect the fact that in reality cancellous bone is in direct contact with the prosthesis. The cement layer will also be hypothesized as having uniform thickness between the prosthesis and bone, and all interfaces will be assumed to be ideal, i.e., they would transmit arbitrarily large tensional and compressive loads across their surface without breaking or sliding.

For all these reasons, the problem is grossly oversimplified; moreover, for the same reasons, we will solve it as a two-dimensional (2D) problem; this though, will help provide a better visualization of the results.

The single steps involved in the analysis will be discussed sequentially; these are: preprocessing (i.e., geometrical modeling and meshing), solution of the discretized equations, and postprocessing. For illustration reasons, we will use ANSYS, one of the first commercial FEM codes available. The reader, though, should bear in mind that there are many equally valid commercial FEM software packages available in the market.

3.3.1
Preprocessing

The first step of the process consists of drawing the component that has to be analyzed. FEM software is not programs specifically designed for drawing purposes, therefore this task is best performed through a solid modeler or CAD; the solid model can then be imported into the FEM software. The example we have chosen is shown in Figure 3.1.

It is important that the geometrical features of the part that has to be analyzed are reproduced with sufficient precision, as the results may be affected by an inaccurate geometrical representation. On the other hand, there are features that are not essential to the analysis we want to perform and can thus be disregarded in the geometrical model, in order to simplify the analysis and obtain the results more quickly. Experience is the main guide in choosing what to draw exactly, and this changes according to the particular component that is being represented. However, as a rule of thumb, the areas that have to be drawn accurately are those that are close to the loading points or to the geometrical constraints, and especially those in the vicinity of material discontinuities. An alternative way of drawing or importing the geometry from CAD software is to obtain the geometry from imaging techniques such as computerized tomography (CT)

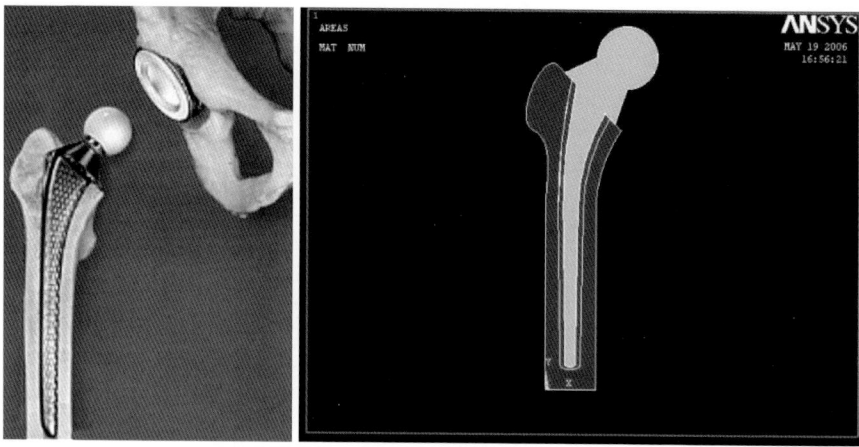

Fig. 3.1 A solid model (*left*) and the geometrical model (*right*) of the sample problem. Each color represents a different material

scans, or from three-dimensional (3D) scanners. These can be used, for example, in the case of a customized simulation, i.e., a patient-specific simulation.

Let us return to our problem and apply the loads. As stated previously, we will define the loading from the acetabular part as a single point force acting vertically on the top of the head of the prosthesis (Fig. 3.2). The bone holding the prosthesis will also have to be constrained in order to simulate that the person is standing. To do this in our example, we will simply define that the lower part of the bone is held fixed, as shown in Figure 3.2. Note that this part of the problem setting, i.e., the imposition of what are called the boundary conditions, is an extremely important part of the problem. The boundary conditions are in fact an integral part of the mathematical model that FEM solves: an erroneous choice of the boundary conditions will lead to incorrect results, irrespective of everything else. In our sample problem, we have chosen boundary conditions driven mainly by simplicity: in doing this, many important features of the problem have been disregarded: the load from the acetabular part is not a point load, but rather a distributed load, and something analogous can be said about the constraint we have applied at the prosthesis base. The choice of the boundary conditions is dictated by the knowledge of the physics of the problem, and is often an issue that is not taken into account properly; it is also a place where the problem can be unduly oversimplified.

The core of the method is the next step, i.e., meshing or discretization. The equations constituting the mathematical model are rewritten in a particular form, called the "weak form". It is beyond the scope of this chapter to describe what a weak form is; suffice it to say that the equations constituting the model will be rewritten in a certain integral form that is suitable to be solved in particular subdomains called "elements". The weak form can be demonstrated to be perfectly equivalent to the starting mathematical model in differential form. To take advantage of this, the whole domain, in our case the hip prosthesis, the proximal femur, and the bone cement, is decomposed into

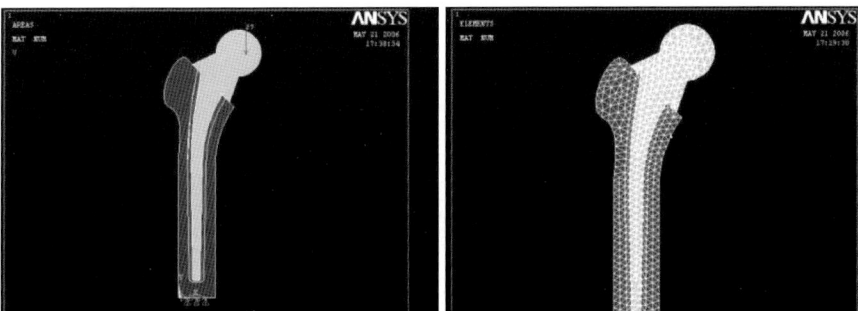

Fig. 3.2 Our sample problem with the boundary conditions (*left*) and a possible mesh (*right*)

a certain number of elements possessing a convenient, simple shape, in our case triangles (Fig. 3.2).

The decomposition of the domain into elements is called a "mesh", and has two purposes: the first is to solve the equations of the mathematical model in a "simple" domain, thus avoiding the complication of dealing with geometrical complexity. Secondly, the decomposition in elements (for example triangular elements) approximates quite well to domains characterized by very complex geometries. This is one of the most interesting features of FEM, one that makes this numerical method particularly attractive in many fields. In fact, other numerical methods work best only in the case of very simply shaped domains, e.g., a rectangular or box-shaped domain; in real-life problems, and particularly in the biomedical fields, one usually can't deal just with boxy domains!

An illustration of possible 2D and 3D elements is given in Figure 3.3. Within the elements there is a certain number of important points, called "nodes", often occupying the vertices of the element, but sometimes also being present in different locations such as the midpoint of an element's edge. The number of nodes in an element is directly related to the accuracy of the solution obtainable from that element. As an example, consider the triangular element in the upper right part of Figure 3.3. The element that is pictured is the one we actually used for our sample problem and, as we can see from the picture, it has six nodes; on the other hand, a triangular element with three nodes at the triangle vertices would also be a possible element, the difference between these two elements being that the one with six nodes will yield more accurate results.

Accuracy is also connected to the total number of elements and, as a consequence, to the total number of nodes that are used in the mesh. The total number of nodes, in particular, is very important because it is exactly in the nodes that the equations constituting the mathematical model are being solved by FEM. Since the equations will be solved in the nodes, having many elements (and thus nodes) will yield a globally more accurate solution. However, the more nodes there are, the more the computer will need time and memory in order to perform its tasks. As a consequence, a finer mesh gives better results but these may take longer and may even require too much memory. Moreover, one should take into account that the elements are also used to approximate

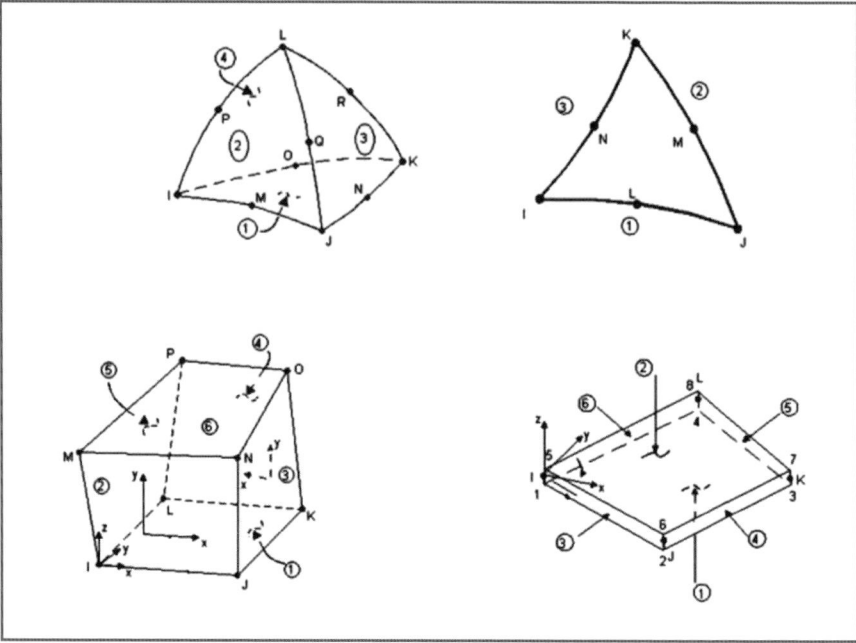

Fig. 3.3 Four typically used elements. Starting from top left, clockwise: a tetrahedral solid element with ten nodes, a planar triangular element with six nodes, a four-node shell element, and an eight-node brick

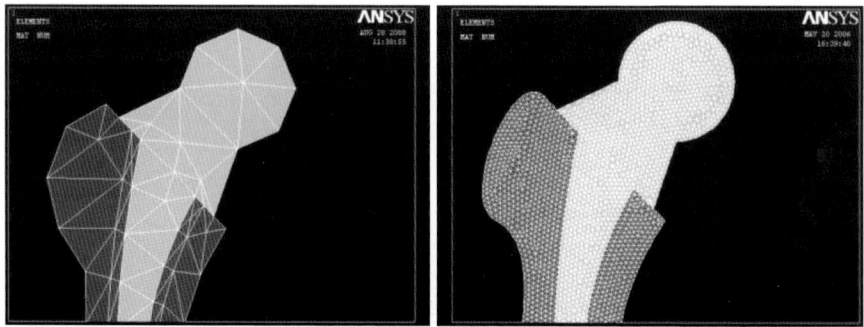

Fig. 3.4 Two limiting mesh choices: a coarse mesh (*left*) and a fine mesh (*right*)

the analysis domain (Fig. 3.4), so a coarser mesh will also imply a poorer domain approximation.

The choice of the mesh is one of the key steps of the whole procedure. Although the results should be mesh independent, it usually isn't so: a bad mesh can in fact spoil an otherwise well-devised FEM analysis. While there can be advantages in choosing the elements as having more or less the same dimensions, the best trade-off is to use mesh refinement, so that more elements (and nodes) can be used only where they are really needed. Again, the choice of a good mesh is mostly a matter of experience; as a rule of thumb, the same guidelines we saw for drawing precision hold also in this case, with the additional note that it is useful to refine the mesh in areas where we are actually seeking the solution. Since we are more interested in finding stresses and strains in bone, it makes sense to refine the mesh here and to leave a coarser mesh in the prosthesis head (Fig. 3.5), even if the load application point is there. This feature will allow us to obtain an accurate solution at the points we are interested in, without wasting too much time and computer resources.

Let us now come to the mathematical model. Its importance is secondary only to the choice of boundary conditions. In our case, the equations that FEM will solve numerically are the balance of linear momentum, i.e., the equivalent of Newton's second law of dynamics, specified for deformable bodies. There isn't much to argue about their validity, notwithstanding they must apply to the specific materials constituting the bodies of interest through what is called a "constitutive equation", i.e., a mathematical model that describes how a certain material deforms under the effect of external forces. Roughly speaking, it tells us whether a certain material is hard or soft, stiff or compliant. Needless to say, these constitutive equations must be chosen accurately.

In the FEM commercial software available on the market today, the user can simply select the constitutive equation that best suits his needs among the various ones that are already implemented in the software itself. Generally, the most frequently used constitutive equations are built-in in almost all commercial software. Like the boundary conditions, the constitutive equations are a fundamental part of the mathematical model: an improper choice of the constitutive equation will inevitably lead to incorrect results.

In the sample problem we are considering, we will choose for all the materials (the metal of the prosthesis, bone cement, and cortical bone) an isotropic linearly elastic constitutive equation. This is the simplest choice one can make, but of course, in the case of a real problem it may be too simplistic: what we are assuming is first of all that

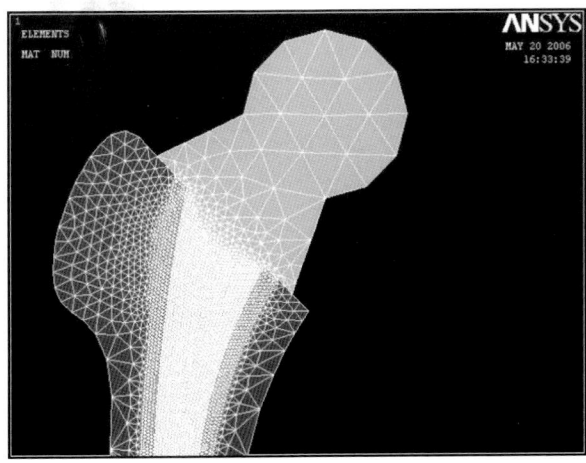

Fig. 3.5 A good choice: a mesh that is refined only at points where it is needed

all the materials are elastic. Elasticity means that the material will deform under a certain load up to its final shape. After the load is removed, the material is supposed to return to its original shape following the same path in reverse. In fact no real material is truly elastic but elasticity may be thought of as a good approximation for many materials (particularly metals), especially if they are subject to small deformations. Usually it is not a good hypothesis for polymers (including the acrylic of bone cement of our sample problem and silicones such as Silastic®) or biological materials, whose behavior is best approximated by a viscoelastic constitutive equation.

Moreover, we have also supposed that the materials are linear. This has two different meanings: from the physical point of view it means that the deformation of the material is proportional to the applied loads, an instance that is often (but not always) verified in real materials at least at small deformations. More importantly, if the constitutive equation is linear, the mathematical problem itself becomes linear, and this guarantees the existence and uniqueness of the solution we are looking for, provided the problem is well posed.

As a further simplification, we have assumed the materials to be isotropic, i.e., their mechanical behavior is the same irrespective of the direction in which they are loaded. This simplifying hypothesis is never true in a strict sense; nevertheless, for many materials it is acceptable, taking into account the considerable simplification introduced. In the specific case, we can say that the metal of the prosthesis and the bone cement can be thought of as isotropic without committing a significant error. On the other hand, bone, together with almost every natural tissue, is usually strongly anisotropic, its properties varying greatly depending on the loading direction, as a consequence of adaptation and optimization of natural tissues.

In any case, the linearly elastic constitutive equation can be used only if the deformations are very small: this is an intrinsic limitation of the model. In particular, a linearly elastic constitutive equation should not be used if the expected maximum strains exceed 5%. Despite all these problems, the linearly elastic constitutive equation is by far the most widely used constitutive equation, mainly for its simplicity and for the guarantee of obtaining some results through linearity.

As a final point, every constitutive equation has a certain number of parameters that need to be specified. Such parameters are material constants that are normally obtained through experimental measurements. As an example, the constitutive equation we have chosen for our sample problem requires the specification of just two material constants for each material, namely its Young's modulus and Poisson's ratio. The former is a measure of the stiffness of the material and can be obtained directly with a simple tension test. The latter is a measure of the transverse contraction when the material is pulled in the longitudinal direction, also obtainable from the simple tension test. Although both these constants are measured in a particular deformation, i.e., the simple tension experiment, once they are specified it is possible to know the mechanical behavior of an isotropic linearly elastic material for any deformation, provided it is of small entity.

In our sample problem, the values for Young's modulus and Poisson's ratio for each material that is used are listed in Table 3.1. These are common values and are used here only for illustrative purposes.

Table 3.1 Young's modulus and Poisson's ratio for the materials used in our simulation

	AISI 316L prosthesis	Acrylic-based bone cement	Cortical bone
Young's modulus (MPa)	200,000	1000	10,000
Poisson's ratio	0.35	0.4	0.35

3.3.2
Solution

Once geometry, material properties, and external loads and constraints are specified, and after the domain has been meshed, the computer can start calculating the solution. It is not within the scope of this chapter to elucidate all the steps involved in the numerical solution; nevertheless, the interested reader should know that the starting differential equations, which were put in weak form during meshing, are now transformed into a reasonably large set of algebraic equations, and are now treatable from the numeric point of view. Moreover, if the mathematical model is linear, these algebraic equations constitute a linear system of equations with the same number of equations as unknowns, and this number is directly proportional to the number of nodes of the mesh. It is exactly for this reason that, as we noted earlier, if the problem is well posed in terms of boundary conditions, the computer will inevitably find the solution to the problem.

If the mathematical model is non-linear, unfortunately there is no general direct solving method known to man, therefore the strategy that is followed is to linearize the problem, i.e., roughly speaking, to divide the general problem into a sequence of smaller steps. In each of these steps, a linear problem that is locally equivalent to the general problem can be solved, so that the general solution can be reconstructed with a step-by-step procedure, but with a sort of trial and error scheme that is not guaranteed to converge. This is indeed the hardest part in running a non-linear analysis. Unlike a linear analysis, the computer here may not be able to find any solution to the problem, even if the problem is well posed. Here the difficulty is related to the problem itself and may be resolved sometimes by writing a finite element code that is specific for the problem at hand, thus not relying on a general-purpose commercial FEM software package. Such a way of proceeding requires, of course, a good familiarity with the mathematics of the finite element method, time and, most of all, a great capacity for dealing with computers without getting frustrated.

3.3.3
Postprocessing

Once all the algebraic equations are solved, the results are ready to be displayed. This can be done in tabular or graphic form; the latter is the most common. As an example, in Figure 3.6 the table with the calculated displacements at the nodes is pictured (left panel). In the panel on the right, the same information is displayed in graphical form through a contour plot. Usually this is a color scale, with colors tending towards yellow and red meaning higher values, and colors like blue and green meaning lower values. In Figure 3.6 the contour plot is in grayscale; therefore higher values correspond to light gray, while lower values correspond to dark gray or black. As expected, the displacement is maximum close to the prosthesis head (light gray), while the basis of the assembly bone-prosthesis, which was held fixed through the geometrical constraint, has zero displacement (black). Note that in our problem the displacements are very small, the maximum displacement being slightly below 0.25 mm.

Interestingly, in the graphical representation the results of interest are displayed at every point of the domain, even if, as we said before, the equations are solved only at the nodes. In the case of FEM, in fact, the results at the nodes can be used to also approximate the quantities of interest at different points from the nodes, through interpolation. This makes FEM a very powerful method: no experimental method is able to calculate the quantities of interest at every point of the body. This means also, though, that even if results are available at every point, the most accurate quantities are calculated at the nodes; thus if one is interested in calculating results at a particular location, the mesh should be structured in such a way that a node is placed at that location.

Let us now be a little more precise about Figure 3.6: the displacement is a vector; therefore, as can be seen from the left panel of Figure 3.6, it has three components that are listed in the table, UX, UY and UZ, but, since we have adopted a 2D analysis, the third component (UZ) is zero for every node. Regarding the graphical representation, since vectors cannot be easily represented in a figure, the vector magnitude, which is a scalar, is displayed. This is also listed in the table as "USUM".

In fact, the graphical representation is rarely used for quantities that are not scalar, i.e., quantities that are identified simply by a number. This is particularly significant

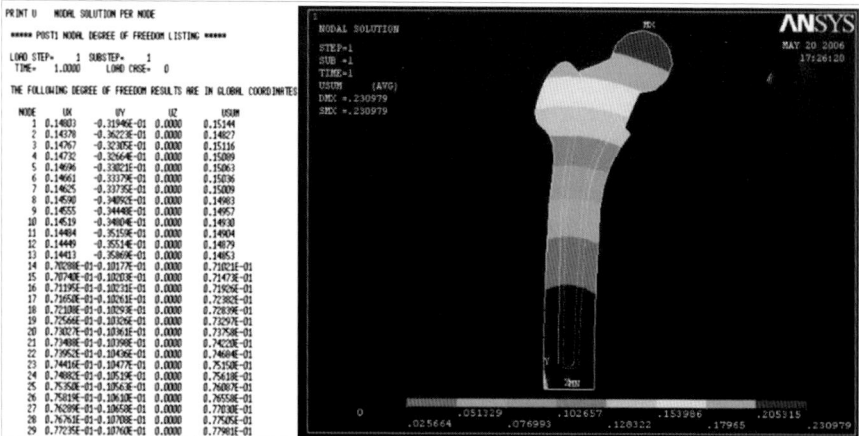

Fig.3.6 A part of the tabular representation of the displacement results at the nodes (*left*) and its graphical representation (*right*)

when the quantity to be represented is stress: stress is a tensorial quantity, i.e., a quantity that is even more general than a vector. In general, a symmetric tensor, such as the stress σ, has six independent components, σ_{xx}, σ_{xy}, σ_{xz}, σ_{yy}, σ_{yz}, and σ_{zz}, and can be represented as a square matrix:

$$\sigma = \begin{bmatrix} \sigma_{xx} & \sigma_{xy} & \sigma_{xz} \\ \sigma_{xy} & \sigma_{yy} & \sigma_{yz} \\ \sigma_{xz} & \sigma_{yz} & \sigma_{zz} \end{bmatrix}$$

In order to visualize stress with a contour plot, such as the ones of Figure 3.7, one can either plot separately the six individual components of stress, or use a suitable scalar measure of stress. The latter is the most common choice, and the measure that is most commonly used (or actually misused) is the "von Mises equivalent stress":

$$\sigma_e = \frac{1}{\sqrt{2}} \sqrt{(\sigma_{yy} - \sigma_{zz})^2 + (\sigma_{zz} - \sigma_{xx})^2 + (\sigma_{xx} - \sigma_{yy})^2 + 6(\sigma_{xy}^2 + \sigma_{xz}^2 + \sigma_{yz}^2)}$$

This quantity has physical meaning only for metals such as steel. In particular, it can be shown that σ_e is related to the distortional elastic energy that leads isotropic metals to yielding when loaded in a general way. Although σ_e is meaningful only if one is interested in the yield point of metals, it is often used also in the case of different materials, due to ignorance about what the von Mises stress really is and the fact that a convenient quantity such as σ_e does not exist for other materials. In any case, even if the use of σ_e can be tolerated for certain materials other than metals, it should definitely not be used in the case of anisotropic materials (even anisotropic metals), where it really has no meaning whatsoever.

Turning back to our sample problem, though, we will use the von Mises stress as a stress measure. Remember that all the materials we chose are assumed to be isotropic. The contour plots of the von Mises equivalent stress are illustrated in Figure 3.7 for the prosthesis and for bone. As we can see, the metallic prosthesis has stress values that are one order of magnitude higher than the stress values within bone. This is a consequence of the greater stiffness of the metal of the prosthesis with respect to bone. Despite this, the level of stress in the prosthesis in this case is still very safe, as the yield point of most metals is much higher than the values displayed in Figure 3.7. The region that is more stressed is the bend in the prosthesis stem, as is to be expected due to the flexural loading acting in this area.

Concerning bone (right panel of Fig. 3.7), the area that is mostly loaded is the bottom part, while the top regions, especially close to the greater trochanter, are basically stress free. This in part justifies our choice not to draw or mesh the top regions in any detail, since they contribute little to the overall stress of the geometric model. The fact that the maximum stress is reached in the bottom part is a consequence of the geometrical constraint that was superimposed, together with the stiffness of the metallic stem: this aspect, together with the higher stresses in the stem with respect to bone, are the effects of the well-known stress-shielding phenomenon, that appears even in our oversimplified example.

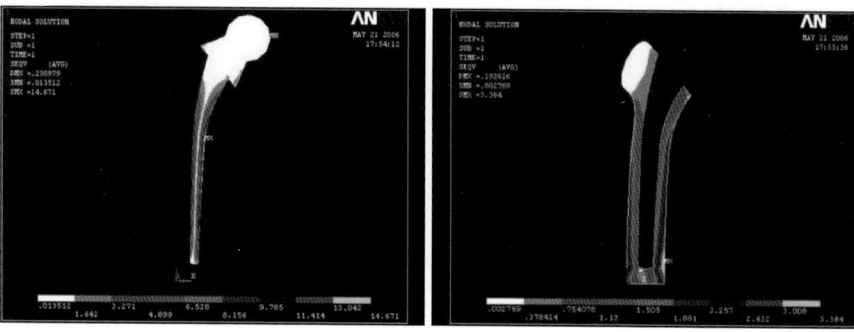

Fig. 3.7 Stress distribution in the prosthesis stem (*left*) and in bone (*right*)

3.4
Conclusions

In this chapter the finite element method has been introduced by using a sample problem in order to describe a typical sequence of operations. The interesting aspects of this numerical method are that it is also easily applicable to complex geometries and that the solutions of interest can be calculated at every point of the geometrical domain.

FEM by itself, though, does not solve the problem: as was stated early in the chapter, the method is merely a numerical procedure that can be used to solve a set of differential equations; it is the responsibility of the FEM user to choose the correct differential equations to solve. Moreover, FEM needs as input a certain number of quantities, such as material parameters or boundary conditions, which have to be measured through a suitable experimental procedure.

This is indeed a very important point: FEM, i.e., a theoretical/numerical way to estimate the solution to a given problem, always needs the input of a certain number of quantities that are obtained from experiments. On the other hand, there is no experimental technique that is capable of obtaining a solution pointwise, e.g., the temperature distribution in a given body or the displacement map of a certain mechanical part. Therefore it is correct to say that FEM and experimental techniques complement each other in achieving the solution to a problem.

Further Reading

Bathe KJ (2007) Finite Element Procedures. Prentice–Hall, Englewood Cliffs, New Jersey.

Belytschko T, Liu WK, Moran B (2000) Nonlinear Finite Elements for Continua and Structures. Wiley and Sons, New York.

Bonet J, Wood RD (1997) Nonlinear Continuum Mechanics for Finite Element Analysis. Cambridge University Press, Cambridge.

Crisfield MA (1996) Non-Linear Finite Element Analysis of Solids and Structures, Vols 1 and 2. Wiley and Sons, Chichester.

Fish J, Belytschko T (2007) A First Course in Finite Elements. Wiley and Sons, New York.

Hughes TJR (2000) The Finite Element Method: Linear Static and Dynamic Finite Element Analysis. Dover, Mineola, New York.

Oden JT (2006) Finite Elements of Nonlinear Continua. McGraw-Hill, New York.

Ratner BD, Hoffman AS, Schoen FJ, Lemons JE (2004) Biomaterials Science, pp 32–34, Elsevier, San Diego, California.

Reddy JN (1993) An Introduction to the Finite Element Method. McGraw Hill, New York.

Reddy JN (2004) An Introduction to Non Linear Finite Element Analysis. Oxford University Press, Oxford.

Simo JC, Hughes TJR (2000) Computational Inelasticity. Springer-Verlag, New York.

Zienkiewicz OC, Taylor RL (2000) Finite Element Method: Vol 1 The Basis. Butterworth Heinemann, Oxford.

Zienkiewicz OC, Taylor RL (2000) Finite Element Method: Vol 2 Solid Mechanics. Butterworth Heinemann, Oxford.

Zienkiewicz OC, Taylor RL (2000) Finite Element Method: Vol. 3 Fluid Mechanics. Butterworth Heinemann, Oxford.

Prostheses for the Joints of the Hand

4

A. Merolli

Abstract Whenever a degenerative, inflammatory or destructive process leads to the complete loss of joint surfaces and morphology, there is an indication for an artificial replacement. For several joints of the hand, the causes that lead to artificial replacement are the same as those encountered in places like the hip or the knee; however, hand joints bear a limited load in comparison, and so alternative surgical procedures to prosthetic replacement, such as, for example, joint fusion, are still good options in many cases. Prostheses for the joints of the hand are reviewed. In principle, an artificial replacement that restores morphology, function and strength may be desirable in many instances but, as we shall see, a good solution still does not exist for hand joints.

Keywords Hand Joints • Metacarpophalangeal Joint • Prostheses • Rheumatoid Arthritis

4.1
Introduction

Whenever a degenerative, inflammatory or destructive process leads to the complete loss of joint surfaces and morphology, there is an indication for an artificial replacement. For several joints of the hand, the causes that lead to artificial replacement are the same as those encountered in places like the hip or the knee.

Artificial replacement of the metacarpophalangeal joints dates back to the 1950s, but it has not become as successful and widespread as, for example, artificial replacement of the hip joint where, today, prostheses have virtually supplanted any other kind of surgery performed in the past.

Hand joints bear a limited load in comparison to the hip or knee, and alternative surgical procedures to prosthetic replacement, such as, for example, joint fusion, are still good options in many cases.

In principle, an artificial replacement that restores morphology, function and strength may be desirable in many instances but, as we shall see, a good solution still does not exists for joints of the hand.

A. Merolli (✉)
Orthopaedics and Hand Surgery, The Catholic University School of Medicine, Rome, Italy

A. Merolli, T.J. Joyce (eds), *Biomaterials in Hand Surgery.*
© Springer-Verlag Italia 2009

4.2
Arthrosis and Arthritis

A common pathological condition which may result in complete destruction and disappearance of the articular cartilage, and painful contact between underlying bone ends, is "osteoarthrosis". This is a degenerative chronic non-inflammatory bone disease (hence the suffix "-osis"), whose mechanism of action is not yet fully understood, but it is recognised that excessive and repeated mechanical overload of the joint does play a part [1]. The disease affects all the joints but it is particularly severe in larger weight-bearing joints of the lower limb, like the hip and the knee.

The terms "osteoarthrosis" and "osteoarthritis" are found in broad use and with a certain degree of overlap in the orthopedic literature [2].

The term "osteoarthritis" should be reserved, more appropriately, for those conditions where inflammation is the primary cause of articular damage. Rheumatoid arthritis is the most common osteoarthritis affecting the hand joints (Fig. 4.1); it is a severe disease that may damage several tissues and areas in the body and, when a joint is involved, may lead to a total loss of articular cartilage coupled with gross deformity of the joint ends, producing a painful and debilitating condition which can require an artificial joint replacement.

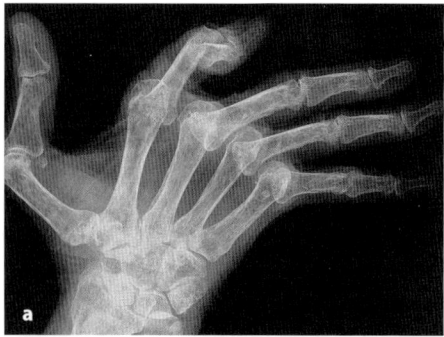
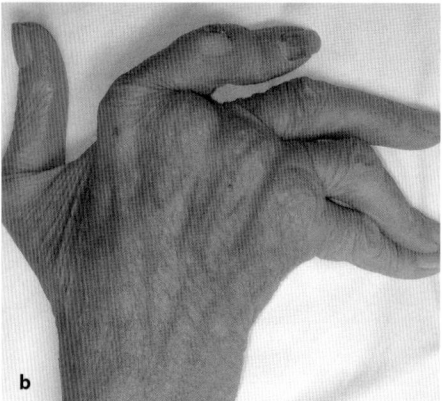

Fig. 4.1 Rheumatoid arthritis is the most common osteoarthritis affecting the hand joints; it may lead to a gross deformity because of partial volar dislocation of the metacarpophalangeal joints and ulnar drift of the fingers (**a**), resulting in a painful and debilitating condition for the patient (**b**)

4.3
Metacarpophalangeal Joint Prostheses

The metacarpophalangeal (MCP) joint plays a unique role in hand function, as, even if all the other hand joints are immobilized, it is possible to maintain a prehensile function with the sole action of the MCP joints.

In the late 1950s, a tentative prosthetic replacement was described by Brannon and Klein [3]. Since their prosthesis, more than 20 designs have been proposed that have reached a clinical application. In the vast majority of cases these prostheses have been short-lived and are no longer in use or in production [4–7].

Rheumatoid arthritis is by far the principal indication for a MCP joint replacement but, at the same time, the most difficult to address successfully. Better results have been obtained when the cause of joint destruction was a crushing trauma or a degenerative bone disease (osteoarthrosis).

More than 40 years' history tell us that there is not yet any successful design for prosthetic replacement of the MCP joint that is able to simultaneously relieve pain, restore cosmetic appearance, and allow a load-bearing capacity.

Early simplification in design was partly responsible for the initial failures. First, the complex biomechanics of the MCP joint were too simplistically reduced to a cylindrical hinge. Secondly, the stability of the stems relied on polymethyl-metacrylate bone cement (although some designs were proposed with the possibility of a dual cemented–cementless implantation) and failure of the cement was experienced in a significant number of cases. Thirdly, the same design was quite often used for MCP and for proximal interphalangeal (PIP) or distal interphalangeal (DIP) prosthetic replacement, resulting in mixed results for the clinical outcome, which was often better for the PIP and DIP implants mostly used in osteoarthrosis, than for the MCP implants mostly used in rheumatoid arthritis.

The high rigidity of the very early designs led to implant loosening due to bone rarefaction, according to the laws of Wolff and Pauwels [8, 9]; for this reason, the design by Swanson of a single-piece all-flexible prosthesis made of silicone elastomer was a breakthrough [10]. The Swanson design is still the most implanted and most successful, and represents the standard reference in MCP prosthetic replacement. It is successful in relieving pain, improving cosmetic appearance, and simplifying surgical technique (Fig. 4.2), and it is forgiving of failure or breakage of the implant (the patient may still maintain an acceptable MCP function with a broken implant if an adequate peri-implant fibrotic capsule has formed). However, it does not allow the mechanical load that is often necessary for simple activities of daily living.

Developments in MCP designs have not followed a single coherent path; on the contrary, sometimes old errors have been repeated in new designs while good solutions have not been retained in newer models. There is a vast number of papers and several reviews [11–60] in the literature; a step-by-step account is presented in this chapter for teaching purposes.

The early designs were cylindrical hinged rigid metallic prostheses made of two

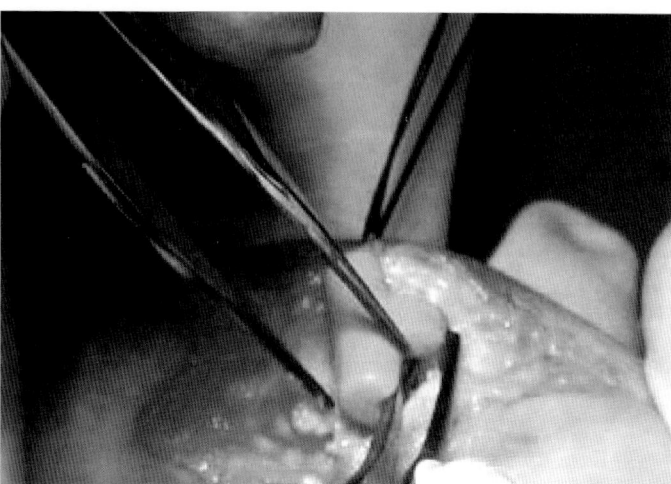

Fig. 4.2 The Swanson design represents the standard reference in metacarpophalangeal prosthetic replacement; the surgical technique is quite simple but the single-piece flexible prosthesis needs to be bent at nearly 180° to be inserted

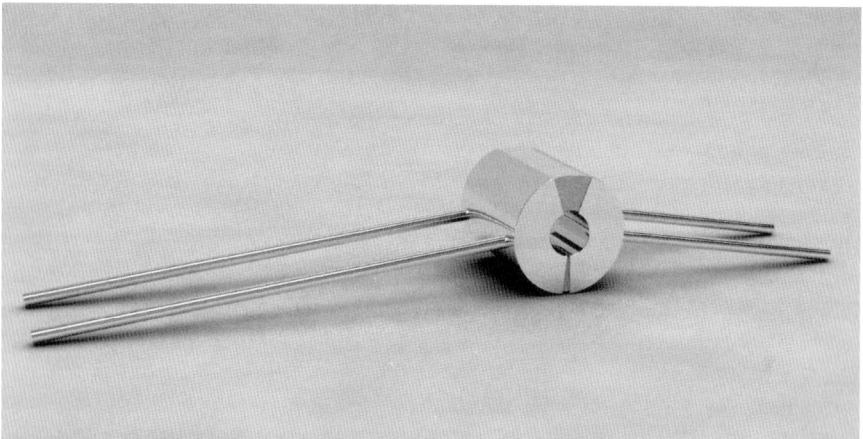

Fig. 4.3 Early designs of metacarpophalangeal joint prostheses were cylindrical, hinged, rigid metallic devices whose components were assembled by the manufacturer; this scheme resembles the Flatt's prosthesis

or more components assembled by the manufacturer (Fig. 4.3). Beevers and Seedhom, in their classification [5], classified these designs as "hinged prostheses".

To reduce rigidity, polyethylene (PE) was soon introduced in the articulation mechanism and often replaced at least one stem (Figs. 4.4 and 4.5). The coupling of metal and PE was (and is) very popular (as it is successfully applied in other areas, such as the hip and knee).

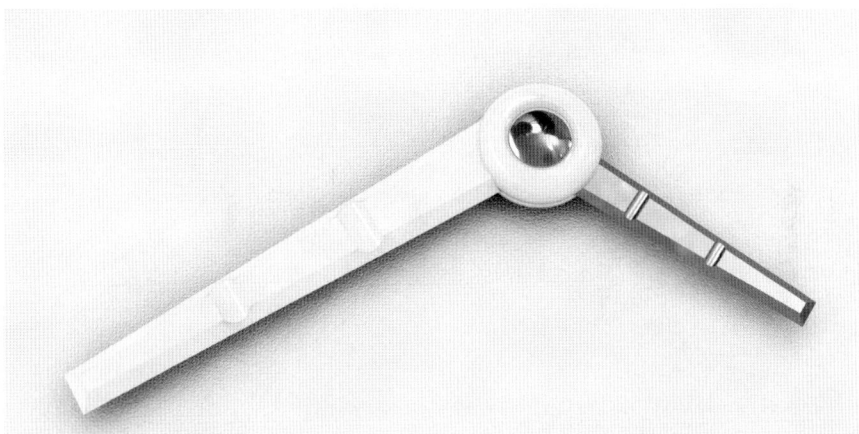

Fig. 4.4 To reduce rigidity, polyethylene (PE) was soon introduced in the articulation mechanism and it often replaced at least one stem, as shown in this scheme which resembles the St George Bucholtz (early design) with a fitting metal–polyethylene hinge

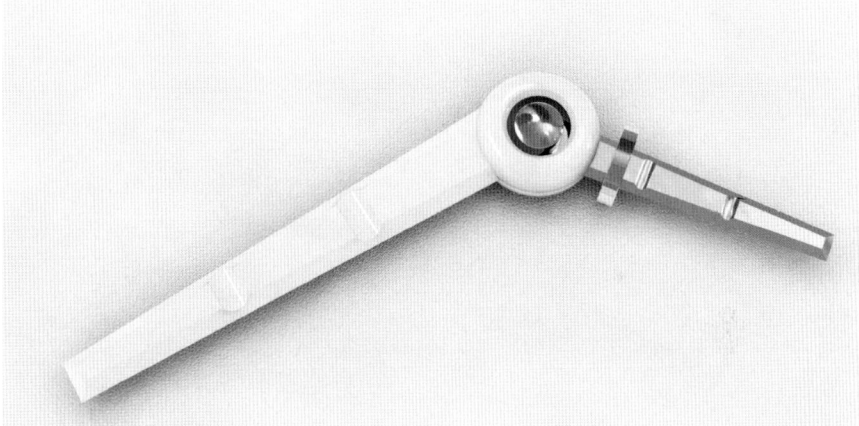

Fig. 4.5 Loosening the fit of the hinge was a way to better adapt to the complex metacarpophalangeal biomechanics; this scheme is for descriptive purposes and does not resemble any design in particular

A better appreciation of MCP joint biomechanics led to designs that took greater account of the anatomical centre of rotation of the joint and the morphology of the phalangeal and metacarpal bone canals (Figs. 4.6 and 4.7).

As has already been stated, the move to a flexible implant resulted in the Swanson design (Fig. 4.8).

Other flexible designs have been proposed, which are closely related to the original Swanson design (they are classified by Beevers and Seedhom as "flexible prostheses"). Improvements have been achieved mostly in perfecting the silicone blend.

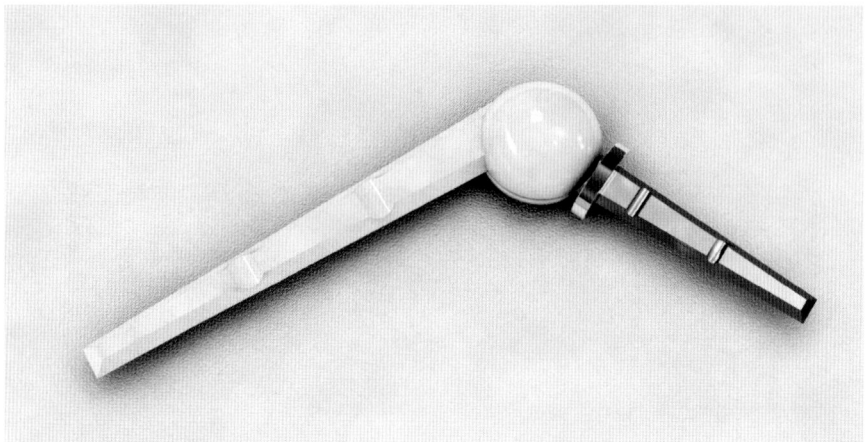

Fig. 4.6 A better appreciation of MCP joint biomechanics led to designs that took greater account of the anatomical centre of rotation of the joint and the morphology of the phalangeal and metacarpal bone canals; the scheme resembles the St Georg prosthesis (late design)

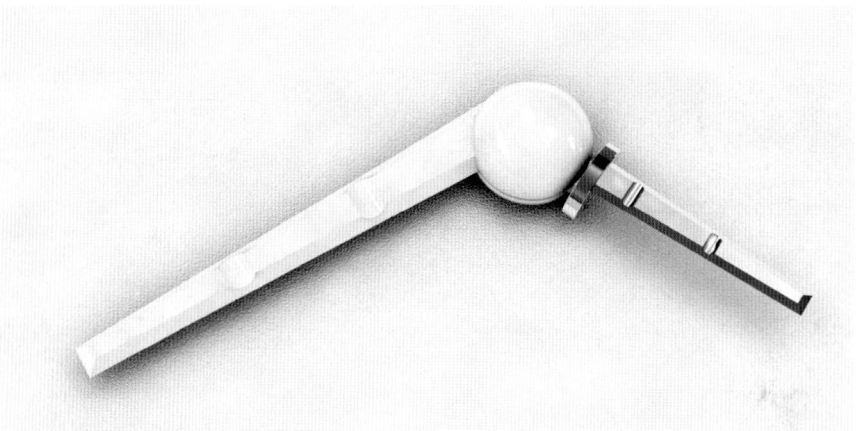

Fig. 4.7 This scheme resembles those designs, such as, for example, the Steffee's, where a more physiological centre of rotation was associated with a better location of the anatomical axes for the metacarpal and the phalangeal bone

An innovation was the pre-flexed design, which aimed to better reproduce the usual position of the MCP joint at rest (Fig. 4.9).

Despite the clinical success of the Swanson, research on "hinged prostheses" was never abandoned, and designs that aimed to better cope with the biological response at the bone–stem interface were produced (Fig. 4.10).

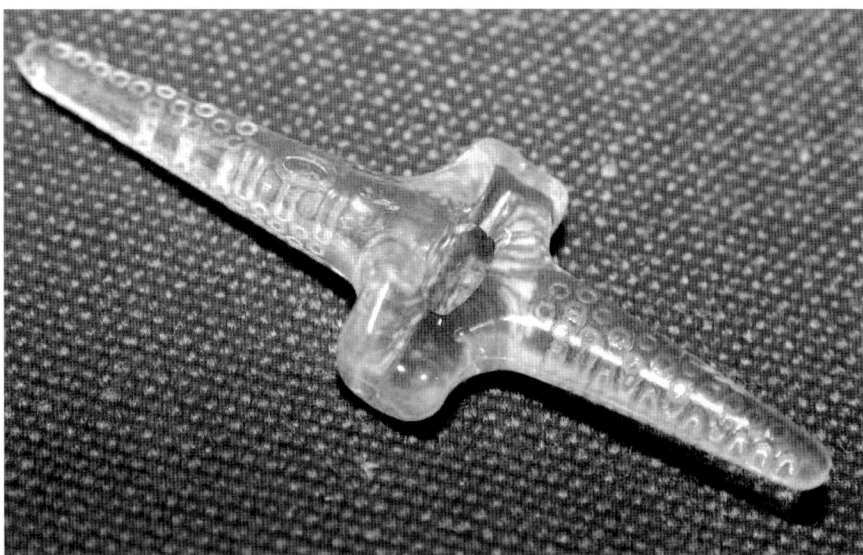

Fig.4.8 An *ex vivo* retrieval of a Swanson prosthesis in which very little superficial wear can be seen, despite its 12 years in service *in vivo*

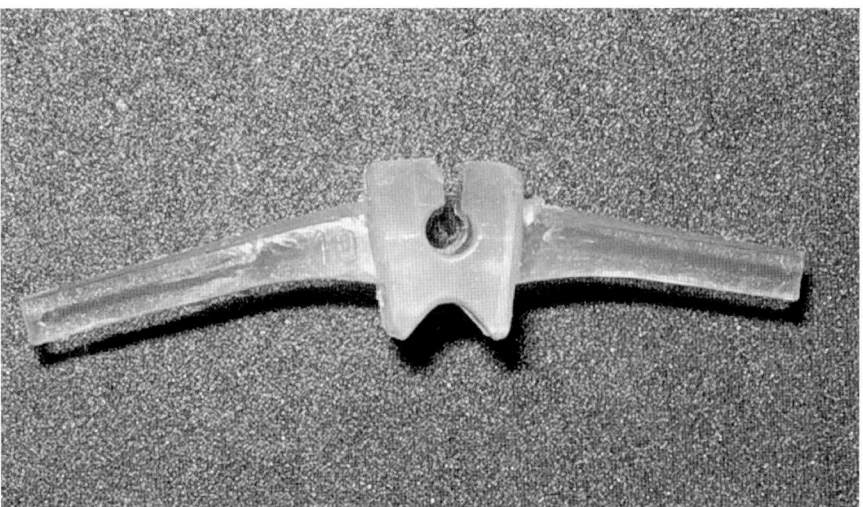

Fig.4.9 An innovation for flexible prostheses was the pre-flexed design

Beevers and Seedhom grouped more recent designs of the 1980s and early 1990s under the term "surface prostheses" and highlight the hybrid presence of characteristics of "hinged" and "flexible" designs. This new class of prosthetic designs grew in number and can be classified as "surface replacement prostheses" (Figs. 4.11 and 4.12).

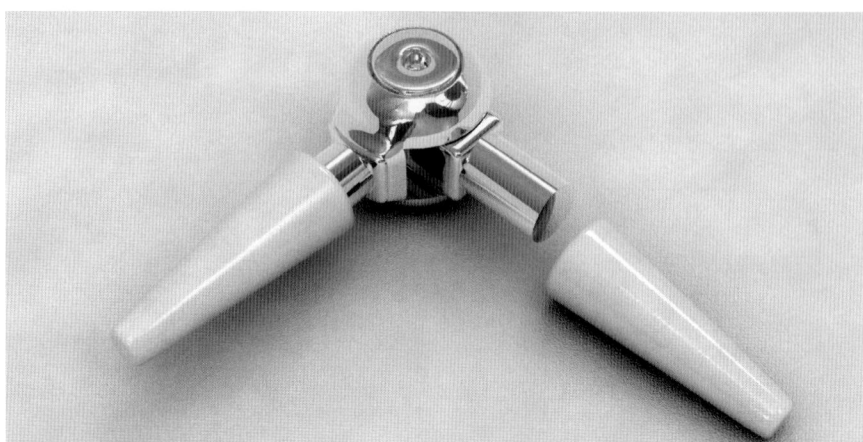

Fig. 4.10 Newer designs of "hinged prosthesis" were intended also to better cope with the biological response at the bone–stem interface; this scheme resembles a Wecko prosthesis, whose stems promoted osteointegration while allowing the sliding of two connecting pistons of the hinge articulation

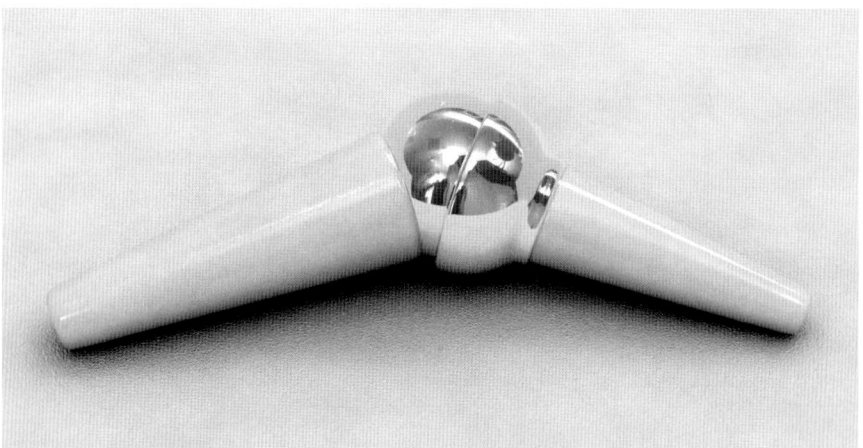

Fig. 4.11 Members of a new class of prosthetic designs grew in number and can be classified as "surface replacement prostheses"; this scheme resembles the Nicolle design

Their technological refinement has been highly remarkable but, unfortunately, most of them (or maybe all) are unsuitable for cases in which joint stability is compromised by severe capsulo-ligamentous destruction, as is often encountered in late stages of rheumatoid arthritis. Therefore, such technological development has failed to address the most difficult indication.

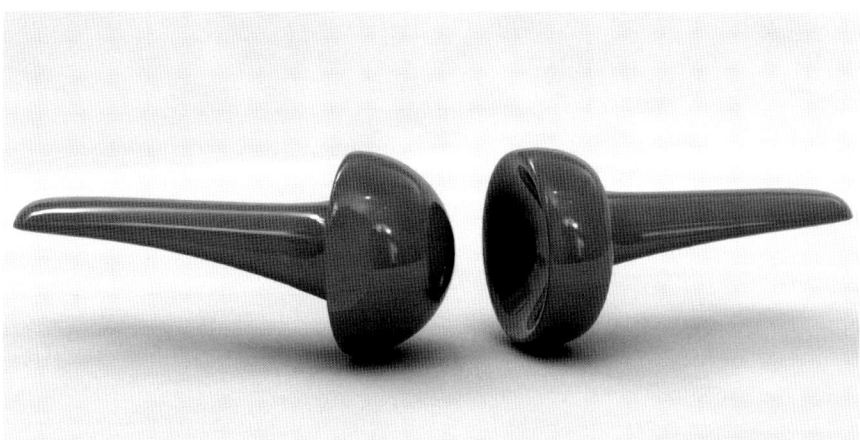

Fig. 4.12 This scheme resembles a pyrolithic-carbon-coated design for surface replacement of the metacarpophalangeal joint

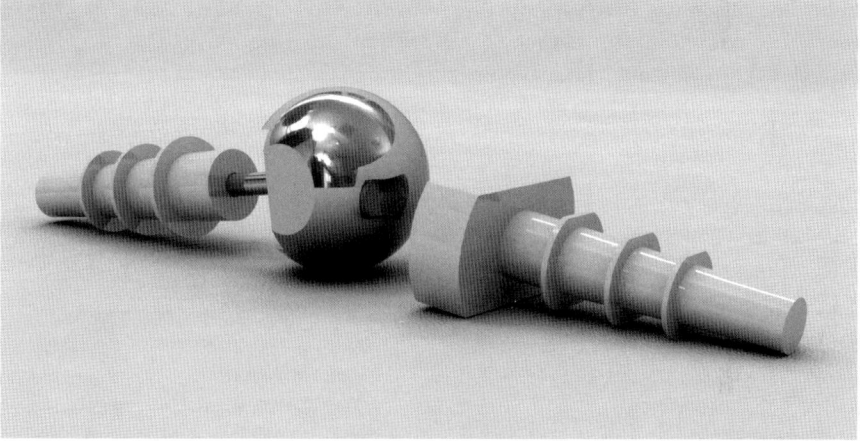

Fig. 4.13 Some designs cannot be classified into the three groups of "hinged", "flexible" or "surface replacement" prostheses. This scheme resembles the Finsbury design, which allows a variable degree of axial rotation and stem pistoning

Some designs cannot be classified into any of these three groups ("hinged"; "flexible"; "surface replacement") but what they share is a kind of piston mechanism for the stems or the articulation, which also allows a variable degree of axial rotation (Fig. 4.13).

As already stated, this history of MCP joint prosthesis development has been presented to help understanding since, in reality, coherent progress did not actually occur. In the author's opinion, there is an opportunity for incorporating various solutions from different designs into a better model; however, research should focus with priority on rheumatoid patients in the later stages of disease – patients who have lost the mechanical competence of capsulo-ligamentous structures. Here, the goal should be to provide a limited but significant load-bearing capacity. Only a successful design addressing this requirement could regain the confidence of both patients and surgeons towards MCP joint prosthetic replacements, reversing the trend which, in the past few years, has seen a steady decrease in the number of implantations performed worldwide and which, in the author's opinion, is only partially related to the progress in medical therapy of rheumatoid arthritis.

4.4
Trapezio-metacarpal Joint Prostheses

While the MCP joint prostheses are, by far, the most important prostheses for the hand joints, both in terms of technological development and clinical demand, many other prostheses have been designed for other parts of the hand, and several have seen a significant clinical application, even if discontinued in some cases.

The second most important joint, which has received much attention and been the focus of clinical studies regarding its replacement with an artificial joint, is the trapezio-metacarpal (TMC) joint or carpal-metacarpal joint I (CMC-I) [61–64]. Like the MCP joint, the TMC joint may be affected by degenerative disease in a significant number of patients. This affliction may lead to complete destruction of the articular cartilage followed by gross alteration of the underlying subchondral bone of the base of the first metacarpal and of the distal articular facet of the trapezium. A clinical and radiographic follow-up may document the progression of this aggressive process, which may have a different duration from patient to patient but generally afflicts subjects for a number of years (Fig. 4.14).

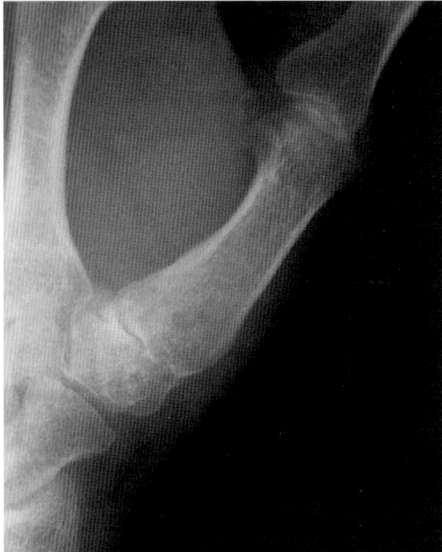

Fig. 4.14 Trapezio-metacarpal degenerative osteoarthrosis may lead to destruction of the articular cartilage and gross alterations of the underlying subchondral bone

An important clinical sign, which should guide the indication for surgical treatment, is pain. In fact, several patients may progress slowly to a complete destruction of the joint, having periods of acute inflammation (which may be controlled by anti-inflammatory drugs) followed by relapses, and never lose an efficient use of the joint (both for working activity and for activities of daily life) because pain is limited and can be kept under control. Other patients, on the other hand, experience an acute debilitating pain which is hardly or not at all eased by drugs while, at the same time, they fail to show any significant damage of joint surfaces on X-ray films.

The degree and control of pain should influence the final decision as to whether or not to propose a surgical procedure. With this view, a conservative treatment may be proposed to patients with extensive destruction but limited pain and no loss of activity, while surgery should be the option for patients with debilitating uncontrollable pain even in the presence of minimal joint destruction.

Several surgical procedures have been proposed for the treatment of TMC joint degeneration or "rhizo-arthrosis". In the author's opinion, "suspension arthroplasty" is among the most effective and a number of techniques have been described. However, several surgeons consider artificial joint arthroplasty a more straightforward surgical procedure and, in some clinical series, recovery after surgery seems to be shorter for artificial arthroplasty in comparison with other techniques.

Several designs have been proposed for the TMC joint arthroplasty [65–104]. The TMC joint is a very complex saddle-shaped joint but its mechanics have been simplified to a ball-and-socket joint in most designs. The ball has been positioned either at the level of the base of the first metacarpal or at the level of the distal articular surface of the trapezium (Fig. 4.15).

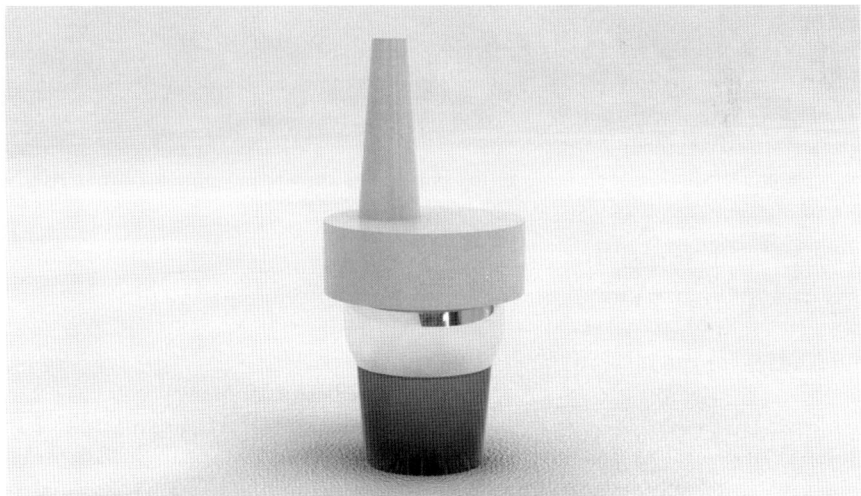

Fig. 4.15 Several designs have been proposed for the TMC joint arthroplasty, simplifying the complex saddle-shaped joint to a ball-and-socket joint; in this scheme, resembling the Mayo TMC prosthesis, the ball has been positioned at the level of the distal articular surface of the trapezium

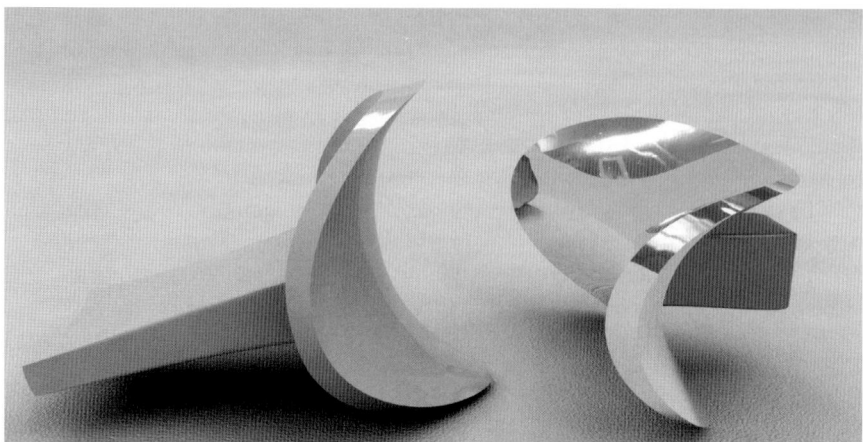

Fig. 4.16 More sophisticated surface replacement joints proposed for the TMC joint arthroplasty better reproduce the anatomy of the natural joint; the scheme resembles the saddle-shaped prosthesis of Linscheid

More recently, more sophisticated surface replacement joints have been marketed which better reproduce the anatomy of the natural joint; saddle-shaped artificial joints have been proposed for the base of the metacarpal bone and for both ends of the joints (Fig. 4.16).

The optimal design may yet be found; the bone–stem interface probably requires better solutions in consideration of the very limited bone stock available. Future designs possibly able to compensate for minor error in positioning will, also, be more welcome in the real surgical setting.

Apart from prostheses, other devices exist that have not been designed as real prosthetic replacements but can be better categorized as "spacers"; these have been proposed and tested clinically. A pyrocarbon-coated disk has been developed as a spacer able to provide a hole by which a suspension tendon arthroplasty may be easily performed. Another recent device is a tissue band made of polycaprolactone-polyurethane, which can be fixed to the bones and aims to promote a fibrous pad in the former joint space.

4.5
Prostheses for the Interphalangeal Joints

While we emphasized that the second joint that has been subject of significant study in terms of prosthetic designs is the trapezio-metacarpal joint, it must be also be noted that a lot of prostheses have been used to substitute damaged distal-interphalangeal (DIP) or proximal-interphalangeal (PIP) joints. However, dedicated studies on DIP and PIP joint designs were very limited for many years, since most of the time surgeons have been happy to simply use smaller versions of designs developed for the MCP joint [105–109]. This fact is linked to the basic simplification of a MCP joint as a cylindrical hinge, while it is, in fact, far more complex. In contrast, DIP and PIP mechanics can be truly exemplified as those of a cylindrical hinge. Several MCP joints have been mistakenly designed as pure cylindrical hinges; in this way they have become more suitable for DIP and PIP joint replacement than MCP joint replacement.

The need for artificial arthroplasty of the DIP and PIP joints is often limited, and cosmetic demands often seem to be more relevant than functional demands. Recent designs purely dedicated to DIP and PIP joints have been proposed to perform a surface replacement (Figs. 4.17 and 4.18); they are unsuitable for MCP joints.

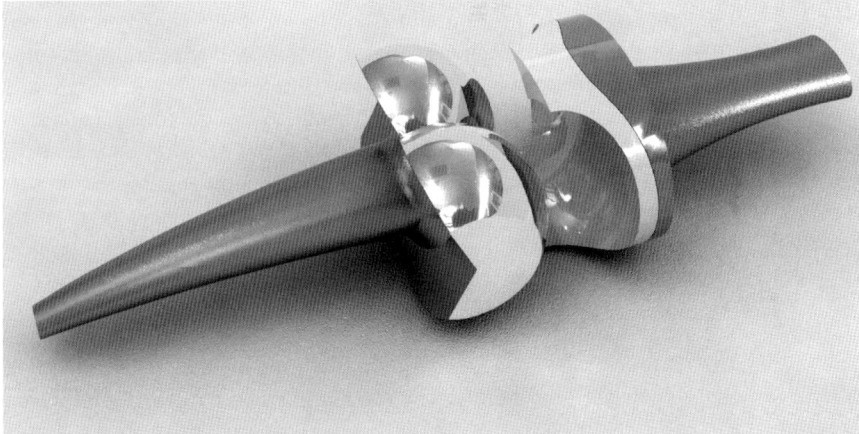

Fig. 4.17 The scheme shows a PIP surface replacement prosthesis with metal-polyethylene articulation and porous coated metallic stems

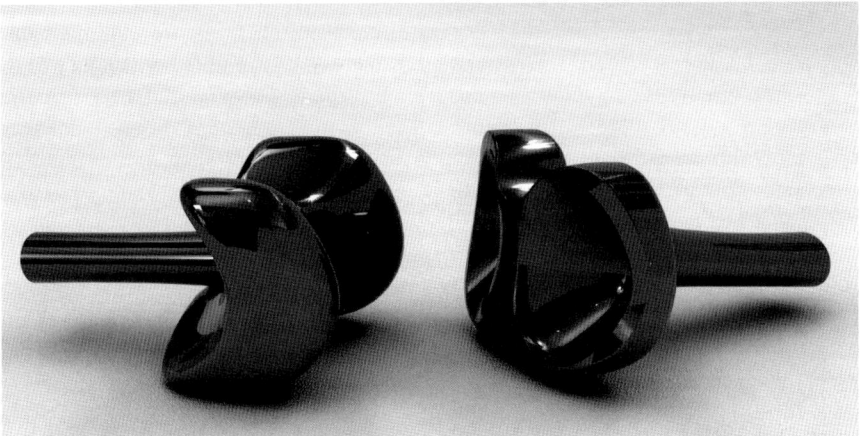

Fig. 4.18 The scheme shows a pyrocarbon-coated prosthesis for PIP surface replacement

They should, however be viewed favorably, because better designs for DIP and PIP joints can lead to an increase in the number of indications for prosthesis implantation of these areas.

4.6
Prostheses for the Scaphoid

Non-united fracture of the scaphoid is still a not-uncommon occurrence. When it is associated with necrosis of the proximal pole it may represent a real challenge for the surgeon and be a debilitating condition for the patient. A simple prosthesis of silicone elastomer was proposed by Swanson. Unfortunately, the excessive load experienced by the implant quickly led to the production of a lot of debris and breakage of the implant. New versions made of mirror-finished titanium alloy or, more recently, of pyrocarbon-coated carbon, have been proposed. There are conflicting reports about these prostheses and they do not seem, at present, to be able to provide a reliable alternative to more traditional surgery such as resection of the proximal carpal row [110–121]. A point that should be emphasized is the continuing progress in surgical treatment of scaphoid fracture, associated with an improvement in its early detection, which could, in the future, result in a decrease in the number of non-united fractures, in turn limiting the need for a reliable prosthetic replacement.

4.7
Prostheses for the Lunate

An artificial lunate has been proposed as a possible treatment for Kienbock's disease.

Kienbock's disease is an isolated disorder of the lunate in which there is progressive collapse of the bone. The cause of Kienbock's disease is unknown and its natural history is uncertain. Various treatments have been suggested for the different stages of the disease. There are two main reasons for this limited knowledge: first, Kienbock's disease is uncommon, so that even a surgeon with a special interest in the hand and wrist will seldom accumulate a large number of personal cases; and secondly, as with osteochondritis or avascular necrosis in other sites, the changes in Kienbock's disease occur slowly so patients must be followed up for many years if a reasonable assessment of the effect of treatment has to be made, and this may not be an easy task.

Total excision of the lunate and its substitution with an artificial replacement has been proposed. Initially, a silicone elastomer prosthesis was proposed, soon replaced by a polished titanium-alloy prosthesis. Clinical results were poor, even if some papers claimed the contrary. More recently, pyrocarbon-coated prostheses have been proposed for this application [122–144].

In the author's opinion, a prosthesis for the lunate may fall into the realm of "devices developed for a ill-posed indication". In fact, it may be a mistake to excise a diseased lunate and replace it with an artificial joint because several surgical treatments seem to be quite effective at maintaining the lunate in place. Techniques of radial shortening, ulnar lengthening, radial decompression and others, have reported good clinical follow-up results, and in some cases a partial restoration of the lunate morphology. As a general rule, the biological structures of the patient should be preserved whenever possible and artificial replacement should be addressed only when there are no better alternatives.

4.8
Mid-carpal Replacement

A prosthesis for the proximal part of the capitate (great bone) has been proposed; in a similar fashion as for scaphoid or lunate prosthesis, it was born as a silicone elastomer device, then was replaced by metallic alloy and nowadays can be found as a pyrocarbon-coated prosthesis (Fig. 4.19).

Indications are limited but there are, nevertheless, cases in which there is no real alternative to providing a surgical option [145].

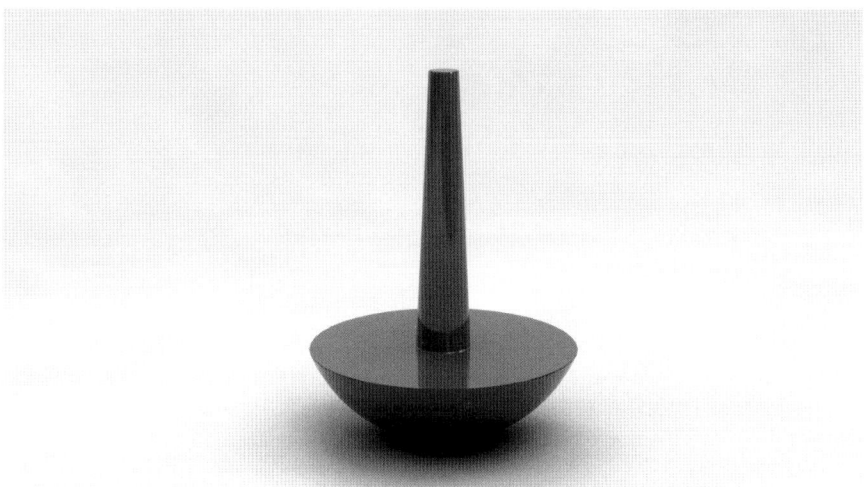

Fig. 4.19 The scheme resembles a pyrocarbon-coated surface replacement prosthesis for the capitate

Acknowledgements
The Author would like to thank Dr. Francesco Scalzitti of RUFA (Rome University of Fine Arts) for his invaluable assistance in producing the 3D drawings of Figures 4.3, 4.4, 4.5, 4.6, 4.7, 4.10, 4.11, 4.12, 4.13, 4.15, 4.16, 4.17, 4.18, and 4.19.

References

1. Dorland's medical dictionary (2007) Elsevier-Saunders, Philadelphia.
2. Stedman's medical dictionary (2007) Lippincott-Raven, Philadelphia.
3. Brannon EW, Klein G (1959) Experience with a finger joint prosthesis. J Bone Joint Surg Am 41A:87–102.
4. Beevers DJ, Seedhom BB (1995) Metacarpophalangeal joint prostheses. A review of the clinical results of past and current designs. J Hand Surg [Br] 20:125–136.
5. Beevers DJ, Seedhom BB (1993) Metacarpophalangeal joint prostheses: a review of past and current designs. Proc Inst Mech Eng 207:195–206.
6. Joyce TJ (2004) Currently available metacarpo-phalangeal prostheses: their design and prospecrtive considerations. Expert Rev Med Device 1:193 – 204.
7. Linscheid RL (2000) Implant arthroplasty of the hand: retrospective and prospective considerations. J Hand Surg [Am] 25:796–816.
8. Wolff J (1986) The law of bone remodelling. Springer-Verlag, Berlin Heidelberg.
9. Pauwels F (1976) Developmental effects of the functional adaptation of bone. Anat Anz 139:213–220.
10. Swanson AB (1968) Silicone rubber implants for replacement of arthritic or destroyed joints in the hand. Surg Clin North Am 48:1113–1127.
11. Adams BD, Blair WF, Shurr DG (1990) Schultz metacarpophalangeal arthroplasty: a long-term follow-up study. J Hand Surg [Am] 15:641–645.
12. Allieu Y, Lussiez B, Martin B (1990) [Long-term results of the Swanson implant for the treatment of basal joint arthrosis.] Rev Chir Orthop Reparatrice Appar Mot 76:437–441.
13. Beckenbaugh RD (1983) Implant arthroplasty in the rheumatoid hand and wrist: current state of the art in the United States. J Hand Surg [Am] 8(5 Pt 2):675–678.
14. Beckenbaugh RD (1983) Preliminary experience with non cemented nonconstrained total joint arthroplasty for the metacarpo-phalangeal joints. Orthopaedics 6:962–965.
15. Beevers DJ, Seedhom BB (1995) Design of a non-constrained, non-cemented, modular, metacarpophalangeal prosthesis. Proc Inst Mech Eng 209:185–195.
16. Bernstein SA, Strickland RW, Lazarus E (1993) Axillary lymphadenopathy due to Swanson implants. J Rheumatol 20:1066–1069.
17. Bieber EJ, Weiland AJ, Volenec-Dowling S (1986) Silicone-rubber implant arthroplasty of the metacarpophalangeal joints for rheumatoid arthritis. J Bone Joint Surg Am 68:206–209.
18. Blair WF, Shurr DG, Buckwalter JA (1984) Metacarpophalangeal joint arthroplasty with a metallic hinged prosthesis. Clin Orthop 184:156–163.
19. Buchler U, Fischer T (1987) Use of a minicondylar plate for metacarpal and phalangeal periarticular injuries. Clin Orthop 214:53–58.
20. Catalano F, Tranquilli Leali P et al (1980) Metacarpo-phalangeal joint. A biomechanic aproach. Acta Orthop Belg 46:678–685.
21. Chung KC, Kowalski CP, Myra Kim H et al (2000) Patient outcomes following Swanson silastic metacarpophalangeal joint arthroplasty in the rheumatoid hand: a systematic overview. J Rheumatol 27:1395–1402.
22. Condamine JL, Benoit JY, Comtet JJ , Aubriot JH (1988) [Proposed digital arthroplasty critical study of the preliminary results.] Ann Chir Main 7:282–297.
23. Cook SD, Beckenbaugh RD, Redondo J et al (1999) Long-term follow-up of pyrolytic carbon metacarpophalangeal implants. J Bone Joint Surg Am 81:635–648.
24. Derkash RS, Niebauer JJ Jr, Lane CS (1986) Long-term follow-up of metacarpal phalangeal arthroplasty with silicone Dacron prostheses. J Hand Surg [Am] 11:553–558.
25. Doi K, Kuwata N, Kawai S (1984) Alumina ceramic finger implants: a preliminary biomaterial and clinical evaluation. J Hand Surg [Am] 9:740–749.

26. Dunkley AB, Leslie IJ (1997) Candida infection of a silicone metacarpophalangeal arthroplasty. J Hand Surg [Br] 22:423–424.

27. El-Gammal TA, Blair WF (1993) Motion after metacarpophalangeal joint reconstruction in rheumatoid disease. J Hand Surg [Am] 18:504–511.

28. Figgie MP, Inglis AE, Sobel M et al (1990) Metacarpal-phalangeal joint arthroplasty of the rheumatoid thumb. J Hand Surg 15A:210–216.

29. Flatt AE (1980) New joints for old. J Hand Surg [Am] 5:525–527.

30. Fleming SG, Hay EL (1984) Metacarpophalangeal joint arthroplasty eleven year follow-up study. J Hand Surg [Br] 9:300–302.

31. Golz R, Kuschner SH, Gellman H (1992) Sequential infection of silicone metacarpophalangeal joint arthroplasties resulting from skin breakdown. J Hand Surg [Am] 17:150–152.

32. Hagert CG, Branemark PI, Albrektsson T et al (1986) Metacarpophalangeal joint replacement with osseointegrated endoprostheses. Scand J Plast Reconstr Surg 20:207–218.

33. Harboldt SL, Gumley GJ, Balogh K (1992) Osteolysis after silicone arthroplasty. Am J Clin Pathol 98:594–597.

34. Harris D, Dias JJ (2003) Five-year results of a new total replacement prosthesis for the finger metacarpo-phalangeal joints. J Hand Surg [Br] 28:432–438.

35. Hollister A, Giurintano DJ, Buford WL et al (1995) The axes of rotation of the thumb interphalangeal and metacarpophalangeal joints. Clin Orthop 320:188–193.

36. Jensen CM, Boeckstyns ME, Kristiansen B (1986) Silastic arthroplasty in rheumatoid MCP-joints. Acta Orthop Scand 57:138–140.

37. Joyce TJ, Milner RH, Unsworth A (2003) A comparision of ex vivo and in vitro sutter metacarpo-phalangeal prostheses. J Hand Surg [Br] 1:86–91.

38. Kay S, Watson JS (1986) Primary flexible implant arthroplasty of the metacarpophalangeal joints during digital replantation. J Hand Surg [Br] 11:414–416.

39. Kirschenbaum D, Schneider LH, Adams DC, Cody RP (1993) Arthroplasty of the metacarpophalangeal joints with use of silicone-rubber implants in patients who have rheumatoid arthritis. Long-term results. J Bone Joint Surg Am 75:3–12.

40. Levack B, Stewart HD, Flierenga H, Helal B (1987) Metacarpo-phalangeal joint replacement with a new prosthesis: description and preliminary results of treatment with the Helal flap joint. J Hand Surg [Br] 12:377–381.

41. Lundborg G, Branemark PI, Carlsson I (1993) Metacarpophalangeal joint arthroplasty based on the osseointegration concept. J Hand Surg [Br] 18:693–703.

42. McArthur PA, Milner RH (1998) A prospective randomized comparison of Sutter and Swanson silastic spacers. J Hand Surg [Br] 23:574–577.

43. McGovern RM, Shin AY, Beckenbaugh RD, Linscheid RL (2001) Long-term results of cemented Steffee arthroplasty of the thumb metacarpophalangeal joint. J Hand Surg [Am] 26:115–122.

44. Nalebuff EA (1984) The rheumatoid hand. Reflections on metacarpophalangeal arthroplasty. Clin Orthop 182:150–159.

45. Pereira JA, Belcher HJ (2001) A comparison of metacarpophalangeal joint silastic arthroplasty with or without crossed intrinsic transfer. J Hand Surg [Br] 26:229–234.

46. Petrolati M, Abbiati G, Delaria G et al (1999) A new prosthesis for the metacarpophalangeal joint. Study of materials and biomechanics. J Hand Surg [Br] 24:59–63.

47. Rittmeister M, Porsch M, Starker M, Kerschbaumer F (1999) Metacarpophalangeal joint arthroplasty in rheumatoid arthritis: results of Swanson implants and digital joint operative arthroplasty. Arch Orthop Trauma Surg 119:190–194.

48. Rothwell AG, Cragg KJ, O'Neill LB (1997) Hand function following silastic arthroplasty of the metacarpophalangeal joints in the rheumatoid hand. J Hand Surg [Br] 22:90–93.

49. Schmidt K, Willburger R, Ossowski A, Miehlke RK (1999) The effect of the additional use of grommets in silicone implant arthroplasty of the metacarpophalangeal joints. J Hand Surg

[Br] 24:561–564.
50. Stothard J, Thompson AE, Sherris D (1991) Correction of ulnar drift during silastic metacar-po-phalangeal joint arthroplasty. J Hand Surg [Br] 16:61–65.
51. Swanson AB, de Groot-Swanson G (1985) Flexible implant arthroplasty of the digits. Indications, methods and results. Acta Orthop Belg 51:679–698.
52. Swanson AB, Poitevin LA, de Groot Swanson G, Kearney J (1986) Bone remodeling phenomena in flexible implant arthroplasty in the metacarpophalangeal joints. Long-term study. Clin Orthop 205:254–267.
53. Synnott K, Mullett H, Faull H, Kelly EP (2000) Outcome measures following metacarpophalangeal joint replacement. J Hand Surg [Br] 25:601–603.
54. Vahvanen V, Viljakka T (1986) Silicone rubber implant arthroplasty of the metacarpophalangeal joint in rheumatoid arthritis: a follow-up study of 32 patients. J Hand Surg [Am] 11:333–339.
55. Varma SK, Milward TM (1991) The Nicolle finger joint prosthesis: a reappraisal. J Hand Surg [Br] 16:187–190.
56. Wanivenhaus A, Lintner F, Wurnig C, Missaghi-Schinzl M (1991) Long-term reaction of the osseous bed around silicone implants. Arch Orthop Trauma Surg 110:146–150.
57. Weightman B, Evans DM, Light D (1983) The laboratory development of a new metacarpophalangeal prosthesis. Hand 15:57–69.
58. Welsh RP, Hastings DE, White R (1982) Resurfacing arthroplasty for the metacarpophalangeal joint. Acta Orthop Belg 48:924–927.
59. Williams NW, Penrose JM, Hose DR (2000) Computer model analysis of the Swanson and Sutter metacarpophalangeal joint implants. J Hand Surg [Br] 25:212–220.
60. Wilson YG, Sykes PJ, Niranjan NS (1993) Long-term follow-up of Swanson's silastic arthroplasty of the metacarpophalangeal joints in rheumatoid arthritis. J Hand Surg [Br] 18:81–91.
61. Eiken O (1971) Prosthetic replacement of the trapezium: technical aspects. Scand J Plast Reconstr Surg 5:131–135.
62. Iselin F, Medina J, Audren JL, Stephan E (1989) Traitement des rhizoarthroses par implants de trapèze en silicone de Swanson. Ann Chir Main 8:230–233.
63. Lehmann O, Herren DB, Simmen BR (1998) Comparison of tendon suspension-interposition and silicon spacers in the treatment of degenerative osteoarthritis of the base of the thumb. Ann Chir Main Memb Super 17:25–30.
64. Badia A (2008) Total joint arthroplasty for the arthritic thumb carpometacarpal joint. Am J Orthop 37(8 Suppl 1):4–7.
65. Adams BD, Unsell RS, McLaughlin P (1990) Niebauer trapeziometacarpal arthroplasty. J Hand Surg [Am] 15(3):487-492.
66. Amadio PC (2005) A comparison of fusion, trapeziectomy, and silastic replacement for the treatment of osteoarthritis of the trapeziometacarpal joint. J Hand Surg [Br] 30(3):331-332.
67. Badia A, Sambandam SN (2006) Total joint arthroplasty in the treatment of advanced stages of thumb carpometacarpal joint osteoarthritis. J Hand Surg [Am] 31(10):1605-1614.
68. Bansal M, Goldman AB, Bullough PG, Mascarenhas B (1992) Case report 706: Silicone-induced reactive synovitis. Skeletal Radiol 21(1):49-51.
69. Bezwada HP, Sauer ST, Hankins ST, Webber JB (2002) Long-term results of trapeziometacarpal silicone arthroplasty. J Hand Surg [Am] 27(3):409-417.
70. Boeckstyns ME, Sinding A, Elholm KT, Rechnagel K (1989) Replacement of the trapeziometacarpal joint with a cemented (Caffiniere) prosthesis. J Hand Surg [Am] 14(1):83-89.
71. Cheze L, Doriot N, Eckert M, Rumelhart C, Comtet JJ (2001) In vivo cinematic study of the trapezometacarpal joint. Chir Main 20(1):23-30.
72. Comtet JJ, Rumelhart C (2001) Total trapezometacarpal prostheses: concepts and classification study. Chir Main 20(1):48-54.
73. Cooney WP 3rd, Leddy TP, Larson DR (2006) Revision of thumb trapeziometacarpal arthro-

plasty. J Hand Surg [Am] 31(2):219-227.

74. Cooney WP, Linscheid RL, Askew LJ (1987) Total arthroplasty of the thumb trapeziometacarpal joint. Clin Orthop Relat Res (220):35-45.

75. de la Caffiniere JY (2001) Longevity factors in total trapezometacarpal prostheses. Chir Main 20(1):63-67.

76. De Smet L, Sioen W, Spaepen D, Van Ransbeeck H (2004) Total joint arthroplasty for osteoarthritis of the thumb basal joint. Acta Orthop Belg 70(1):19-24.

77. Dunaud JL, Moughabghab M, Benaissa S, Vimont E, Degandt A (2001) Rubis 2 trapezometacarpal prosthesis: concept, operative technique. Chir Main 20(1):85-88.

78. Ferrari B, Steffee AD (1986) Trapeziometacarpal total joint replacement using the Steffee prosthesis. J Bone Joint Surg [Am] 68(8):1177-1184.

79. Goldberg I, Amit S, Peylan J, Adler A. (1994) Tendon interposition arthroplasty vs Kessler silicone prosthesis for basal joint arthritis of the thumb. Harefuah 126(12):696-699.

80. Herndon JH (1987) Trapeziometacarpal arthroplasty. A clinical review. Clin Orthop Relat Res (220):99-105.

81. Ho PK, Jacobs JL, Clark GL (1985) Trapezium implant arthroplasty: evaluation of a semiconstrained implant. J Hand Surg [Am] 10(5):654-660.

82. Imaeda T, Cooney WP, Niebur GL, Linscheid RL, An KN (1996) Kinematics of the trapeziometacarpal joint: a biomechanical analysis comparing tendon interposition arthroplasty and total-joint arthroplasty. J Hand Surg [Am] 21(4):544-553.

83. Isselin J (2001) ARPE prosthesis: preliminary results. Chir Mainc20(1):89-92.

84. Lignon J, Friol JP, Chaise F (1990) The history of total trapeziometacarpal prostheses. Ann Chir Main Memb Super 9(3):180-188.

85. MacDermid JC, Roth JH, Rampersaud YR, Bain GI (2003) Trapezial arthroplasty with silicone rubber implantation for advanced osteoarthritis of the trapeziometacarpal joint of the thumb. Can J Surg 46(2):103-310.

86. Martinet X, Belfkira F, Corcella D, Guinard D, Moutet F (2004) Foreign body reaction in osteoarthrosis of the trapeziometacarpal joint treated with trapezectomy and interposition of a Dacron "anchovy". A series of 5 cases. Chir Main 23(1):27-31.

87. Masmejean E, Alnot JY, Chantelot C, Beccari R (2003) Guepar anatomical trapeziometacarpal prosthesis. Chir Main 22(1):30-36.

88. Naidu SH, Kulkarni N, Saunders M (2006) Titanium basal joint arthroplasty: a finite element analysis and clinical study. J Hand Surg [Am] 31(5):760-765.

89. Nicholas RM, Calderwood JW (1992) De la Caffiniere arthroplasty for basal thumb joint osteoarthritis. J Bone Joint Surg [Br] 74(2):309-312.

90. Nilsson A, Liljensten E, Bergstrom C, Sollerman C (2005) Results from a degradable TMC joint Spacer (Artelon) compared with tendon arthroplasty. J Hand Surg [Am] 30(2):380-389.

91. Perez-Ubeda MJ, Garcia-Lopez A, Marco Martinez F, Junyent Vilanova E, Molina Martos M, Lopez-Duran Stern L (2003) Results of the cemented SR trapeziometacarpal prosthesis in the treatment of thumb carpometacarpal osteoarthritis. J Hand Surg [Am] 28(6):917-925.

92. Phaltankar PM, Magnussen PA (2003) Hemiarthroplasty for trapeziometacarpal arthritis - a useful alternative? J Hand Surg [Br] 28(1):80-85.

93. Regnard PJ (2006) Electra trapezio metacarpal prosthesis: results of the first 100 cases. J Hand Surg [Br] 31(6):621-628.

94. Ruffin RA, Rayan GM (2001) Treatment of trapeziometacarpal arthritis with silastic and metallic implant arthroplasty. Hand Clin 17(2):245-253.

95. Schuhl JF (2001) The Roseland prosthesis in the treatment of osteoarthritis. A five years experience with the same surgeon. Chir Main 20(1):75-78.

96. Skytta ET, Belt EA, Kautiainen HJ, Lehtinen JT, Ikavalko M, Maenpaa HM (2005) Use of the de la Caffiniere prosthesis in rheumatoid trapeziometacarpal destruction. J Hand Surg [Br] 30(4):395-400.

97. Sotereanos DG, Taras J, Urbaniak JR (1993) Niebauer trapeziometacarpal arthroplasty: a long-term follow-up. J Hand Surg [Am] 18(4):560-564.
98. Swanson AB, de Groot Swanson G, DeHeer DH, Pierce TD, Randall K, Smith JM, Van Gorp CC (1997) Carpal bone titanium implant arthroplasty. 10 years' experience. Clin Orthop Relat Res (342):46-58.
99. Taylor EJ, Desari K, D'Arcy JC, Bonnici AV (2005) A comparison of fusion, trapeziectomy and silastic replacement for the treatment of osteoarthritis of the trapeziometacarpal joint. J Hand Surg [Br] 30(1):45-49.
100. Teissier J, Gaudin T, Marc T (2001) Problems with the metacarpophalangeal joint in the surgical treatment of osteoarthritis by inserting an ARPE type joint prosthesis. Chir Main 20(1):68-70.
101. Uchiyama S, Cooney WP, Niebur G, An KN, Linscheid RL (1999) Biomechanical analysis of the trapeziometacarpal joint after surface replacement arthroplasty. J Hand Surg [Am] 24(3):483-490.
102. van Cappelle HG, Elzenga P, van Horn JR (1999) Long-term results and loosening analysis of de la Caffiniere replacements of the trapeziometacarpal joint. J Hand Surg [Am] 24(3):476-482.
103. Wachtl SW, Guggenheim PR, Sennwald GR (1998) Cemented and non-cemented replacements of the trapeziometacarpal joint. J Bone Joint Surg [Br] 80(1):121-125.
104. Wachtl SW, Sennwald GR, Ochsner PE, Von Hochstetter AR, Spycher MA (1999) Analysis of two bone-prosthesis interfaces and membranes from non-cemented trapeziometacarpal prostheses. Ann Chir Main Memb Super 18(1):66-72.
105. Nagle DJ, af Ekenstam FW, Lister GD (1989) Immediate silastic arthroplasty for non-salvageable intraarticular phalangeal fractures. Scand J Plast Reconstr Surg Hand Surg 23:47–50.
106. Whalen RL, Bowen MA, Sarrasin MJ, Fukumura F, Harasaki H (1993) A new finger joint prosthesis. ASAIO J 39(3):M480-485.
107. Linscheid RL, Murray PM, Vidal MA, Beckenbaugh RD (1997) Development of a surface replacement arthroplasty for proximal interphalangeal joints. J Hand Surg [Am] 22(2):286-298.
108. Ash HE, Unsworth A (2000) Design of a surface replacement prosthesis for the proximal interphalangeal joint. Proc Inst Mech Eng [H] 214(2):151-163.
109. Uchiyama S, Cooney WP 3rd, Linscheid RL, Niebur G, An KN (2000) Kinematics of the proximal interphalangeal joint of the finger after surface replacement. J Hand Surg [Am] 25(2):305-312.
110. Chaix C, Carlin G, Tonto C, Jouglard JP (1975) Prosthetic replacement of the carpal scaphoid. Rev Chir Orthop Reparatrice Appar Mot 61(Suppl 2):232–235.
111. Egloff DV, Varadi G, Narakas A et al (1993) Silastic implants of the scaphoid and lunate. A long-term clinical study with a mean follow-up of 13 years. J Hand Surg Br 18:687–692.
112. Förster W, Schlegel E (1988) Long-term results of endoprosthetic replacement of the scaphoid bone of the wrist joint. Handchir Mikrochir Plast Chir 20:306–313.
113. Foucher J, Foucher F, Fontaine JL, Herbert A (1972) Acrylic prosthesis of the carpal semilunar and scaphoid bones. 16 cases, indications and results. Chirurgie 98:466–467.
114. Haussman P (2002) Long-term results after silicone prosthesis replacement of the proximal pole of the scaphoid bone in advanced scaphoid nonunion. J Hand Surg Br 27:417–423.
115. Jones KG (1985) Replacement of the proximal portion of the scaphoid with spherical implant for post-traumatic carporadial arthritis. J Hand Surg Br 10:217–226.
116. Pequignot JP, Lussiez B, Allieu Y (2000) A adaptive proximal scaphoid implant. Chir Main 19:276–285.
117. Swanson AB, de Groot Swanson G et al (1997) Carpal bone titanium implant arthroplasty. 10 years' experience. Clin Orthop Relat Res 342:46–58.
118. Swanson AB (1970) Silicone rubber implants for the replacement of the carpal scaphoid and

lunate bones. Orthop Clin North Am 1:299–309.

119. Vidal MA, Linscheid RL, Amadio PC, Dobyns JH (1991) Preiser's disease. Ann Chir Main Memb Super 10:227–235.

120. Viegas SF, Patterson RM, Peterson PD et al (1991) The silicone scaphoid: a biomechanical study. J Hand Surg Am 16:91–97.

121. Wilhelm K (1990) Roentgenological follow-up studies of silicone joint surface replacement in hand surgery as exemplified by scaphoid total and partial prosthesis. Handchir Mikrochir Plast Chir 22:177–182.

122. Alexander AH, Turner MA, Alexander CE, Lichtman DM (1990) Lunate silicone replacement arthroplasty in Kienböck's disease: a long-term follow-up. J Hand Surg Am 15:401–407.

123. Backaert M, Verstreken J, Roex J, Vandekerckhove JR (1985) Long-term results obtained with a silastic lunate prosthesis for Kienböck's disease. Acta Orthop Belg 51:889–896.

124. Barber HM, Goodfellow JW (1974) Acrylic lunate prostheses. A long-term follow-up. J Bone Joint Surg Br 56-B(4):706–711.

125. Eiken O, Necking LE (1984) Lunate implant arthroplasty. Evaluation of 19 patients. Scand J Plast Reconstr Surg 18:247–252.

126. Epping W, Stammer HJ (1990) Late results following endoprosthetic lunate bone replacement. Handchir Mikrochir Plast Chir 22:171–176.

127. Hasselgren G, Jerre R, Ullman M et al (1990) Liquid silicone as a lunate prosthesis. J Hand Surg Br 15:35–39.

128. Jiang W, Ye SX, Wu L (1999) Resection of nerve of wrist combining replacement of lunate with bone cement prosthesis in treatment of Kienbock's disease. Zhongguo Xiu Fu Chong Jian Wai Ke Za Zhi 13:72–74.

129. Kaarela OI, Raatikainen TK, Torniainen PJ (1998) Silicone replacement arthroplasty for Kienböck's disease. J Hand Surg Br 23:735–740.

130. Kato H, Usui M, Minami A (1986) Long-term results of Kienböck's disease treated by excisional arthroplasty with a silicone implant or coiled palmaris longus tendon. J Hand Surg Am 11:645–653.

131. Lagier R (1992) Case report 719. Reaction of synovium and bone to a silicone implant of the lunate. Skeletal Radiol 21:137–139.

132. Lesur E, Merle M, Michon J (1989) Limitations of replacing the semilunar with a Swanson's implant. Rev Chir Orthop Reparatrice Appar Mot 75:281–291.

133. Lichtman DM, Alexander AH, Mack GR, Gunther SF (1982) Kienböck's disease – update on silicone replacement arthroplasty. J Hand Surg Am 7:343–347.

134. Lichtman DM, Mack GR, MacDonald RI et al (1977) Kienböck's disease: the role of silicone replacement arthroplasty. J Bone Joint Surg Am 59:899–908.

135. Merle M, Memeteau D, Michon J (1982) Prosthetic replacement of the semilunar bone. Ann Chir Main 1:253–255.

136. Michon J (1973) Lunarectomy with prosthetic replacement. Rev Chir Orthop Reparatrice Appar Mot 59(Suppl 1):180–186.

137. Oda M, Hashizume H, Miyake T et al (2000) A stress distribution analysis of a ceramic lunate replacement for Kienbock's disease. J Hand Surg Br 25:492–498.

138. O'Flanagan SJ, Curtin J (1992) Lunate silastic arthroplasty in Kienbock's disease. J R Coll Surg Edinb 37:52–56.

139. Pardini AG (1984) Silastic arthroplasty for avascular necrosis of the carpal lunate. Int Orthop 8:223–227.

140. Ramakrishna B, D'Netto DC, Sethu AU (1982) Long-term results of silicone rubber implants for Kienböck's disease. J Bone Joint Surg Br 64:361–363.

141. Swanson AB, de Groot Swanson G (1993) Implant resection arthroplasty in the treatment of Kienböck's disease. Hand Clin 9:483–491.

142. Swanson AB, Maupin BK, de Groot Swanson G et al (1985) Lunate implant resection arthro-

plasty: long-term results. J Hand Surg Am 10(6 Pt 2):1013–1024.
143. Viljakka T, Vastamäki M, Solonen KA, Tallroth K (1987) Silicone implant arthroplasty in Kienböck's disease. Acta Orthop Scand 58:410–414.
144. Wachtl S, Sennwald G, Rodriguez M (1994) Long-term outcome of a silastic semilunar bone prosthesis. Ann Chir Main Memb Super 13:36–41.
145. Milliez PY, Kinh Kha H, Allieu Y, Thomine JM (1991) Idiopathic aseptic osteonecrosis of the capitate bone. Literature review apropos of 3 new cases. Int Orthop 15:85–94.

Causes of Failure in Flexible Metacarpophalangeal Prostheses

5

T.J. Joyce

Abstract Rheumatoid arthritis is a common and debilitating disease which often afflicts the small joints of the hands, especially the metacarpophalangeal joints. Although there have been recent improvements in drug treatments, for a number of patients the final clinical intervention entails the replacement of the natural joint with a prosthesis. The vast majority of such implants are single-piece, flexible, silicone designs. This group includes the Swanson, Sutter and NeuFlex metacarpophalangeal prostheses. The most common mode of failure of these implants is fracture, often at the junction of the distal stem and the hinge. Although such fracture does not always mean that a revision operation is required, it is self-evident that if the fracture rate could be reduced, such implants should provide enhanced results in the hands of patients. A clear way to reduce the fracture rate is to understand how fracture has come about. A cohort of 12 failed and explanted Sutter metacarpophalangeal prostheses were obtained from the hands of three rheumatoid patients. After a macroscopic analysis, the explanted prostheses were sliced so that the fracture faces could be examined under a scanning electron microscope. From the results obtained, a number of features consistent with fatigue failure were identified. These features showed that fracture was initiated on the dorsal aspect of the distal stem and travelled in a palmar–ulnar direction.

Keywords Explant • Fractography • Fracture • Metacarpophalangeal • NeuFlex • Prosthesis • Silicone • Sutter • Swanson

5.1
Introduction

Rheumatoid arthritis is a common inflammatory disease with a prevalence of approximately 1% of the population [1, 2]. This painful and crippling disease is associated with multiple joint involvement, and the small joints of the fingers are most commonly affected [2]. Here the disease causes extreme pain, leads to a severe loss of hand function and results in cosmetically upsetting changes [2, 3]. While the devel-

T.J. Joyce (✉)
School of Mechanical and Systems Engineering, Newcastle University, Newcastle upon Tyne, UK

A. Merolli, T.J. Joyce (eds), *Biomaterials in Hand Surgery.*
© Springer-Verlag Italia 2009

opment of drugs to counteract the effects of rheumatoid arthritis continues [4], in those cases where these drugs are unsuccessful there remains an urgent and, arguably, unmet need for suitable finger prostheses to replace the diseased natural joints. Of the finger joints, the metacarpophalangeal joints are the most important and tend to be replaced far more often than the proximal interphalangeal joints [5].

An extensive range of finger prostheses have been proposed and implanted over the last 50 years, yet the most commonly implanted design remains the Swanson prosthesis, which dates from the 1960s and consists of a single piece of flexible silicone elastomer [6]. It has a central hinge section intended to keep the ends of the finger bones separated, and two stems which fit into holes reamed in the bones on each side of the joint [7]. Such is the importance of the Swanson prosthesis [7–12] that it has been described as the joint replacement of choice for several decades [13]. The Swanson prosthesis is available in 11 sizes and is manufactured from a material known as 'Flexspan', although the manufacturers give few additional material properties. This implant is now supplied with titanium grommets, which slip over the stems and are intended to protect the relatively soft silicone material from damage by bone [14]. The second main design is the Sutter, which is also known as the Avanta [15–19]. More recently, the NeuFlex from De Puy has appeared on the market, and in the UK positive initial clinical results have been reported for this implant in terms of increased flexion in comparison with the Swanson prosthesis [20]. Independent *in vitro* tests have indicated that the NeuFlex design gives greater longevity than the Sutter metacarpophalangeal prosthesis [21]. Other designs of single-piece silicone implants are available too, but are less commonly implanted.

Figure 5.1 shows a Swanson metacarpophalangeal prosthesis above a Sutter metacarpophalangeal prosthesis. As can be seen there are some design differences. For example, the Sutter prosthesis has a larger hinge section and its stems are offset in relation to each other, while the tapered square section stems contrast with the rounded edges of the stems of the Swanson prosthesis.

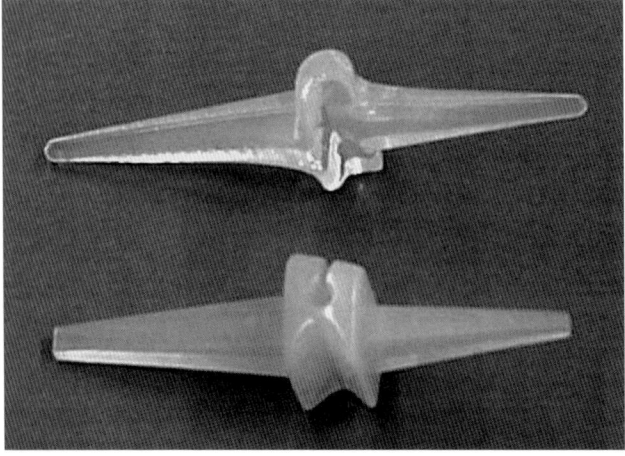

Fig. 5.1 Swanson (*above*) and Sutter (*below*) metacarpophalangeal prostheses

Such has been the success of the Swanson and similar flexible, single-piece silicone designs that they dominate the metacarpophalangeal joint replacement market. Data from the 2008 Norwegian arthroplasty register show that of the 2933 metacarpophalangeal prostheses inserted between 1994 and 2007 in Norway, almost 99% were single-piece flexible designs [5]. The majority (69%) were of the Swanson design, with 22% being supplied by Avanta (Sutter) and the remainder being the newer NeuFlex design [5]. The reason for the dominance of single-piece flexible designs in the metacarpophalangeal joint, replacement market is that such implants, particularly the Swanson metacarpophalangeal prosthesis, have a long history of positive clinical results in terms of achievement of pain relief, improved cosmetic appearance, and a more functional arc of motion. Together, all of these lead to high patient satisfaction [9, 17, 22]. In addition, implantation is relatively straightforward and, should it be necessary, so too is removal.

Despite the dominant position of single-piece silicone implants, there are problems with such devices. These include that they fracture, the body negatively reacts to silicone debris from the implants, and a relatively large amount of bone is removed when surgery is undertaken [8]. In addition, patients tend to show no increase in grip strength or in total range of motion when such implants are fitted [8]. In terms of fracture, it has been shown that approximately two-thirds of such prostheses suffer this fate after 14–17 years in the body [23, 24]. Nevertheless, it should be appreciated that, by the time most of these fractures have occurred, a fibrous tissue pseudojoint has formed, so that, as far as the patient and surgeon are concerned, the finger joint is stable and a revision operation is unnecessary [7]. Therefore, fracture of the implant does not always lead to the need for a revision operation.

Despite this caveat, fracture remains a major concern with flexible metacarpophalangeal prostheses. Figure 5.2 shows a set of Swanson prostheses removed from the hand of one patient. As indicated by the image, fracture generally occurs at the junction of the distal stem and the hinge, a result reported by many hand surgeons [23, 25–28]. This site of fracture is true for both Swanson and Sutter prostheses. As yet, the position of fracture of NeuFlex metacarpophalangeal prostheses does not appear to have been reported in the scientific literature, although a fracture rate of 13% for these implants has been reported at a mean follow-up of 3.6 years [29]. In terms of fracture rates for the Swanson metacarpophalangeal prosthesis, a wide range has been reported [8], the extremes being 0% [30] and 82% [25], both groups at a five-year follow-up. It should also be recognised that fracture can occur at other positions, such as across the hinge and at the junction of the proximal stem and hinge, although these sites of fracture are less commonly seen.

In summary then, fracture of single-piece, flexible silicone metacarpophalangeal prostheses is a major concern. It can lead to a revision operation and therefore 'failure' of the device if revision is defined as the end-point. However, as has also been noted, if fracture occurs but a stable fibrous pseudo-capsule has formed, then a revision operation will generally not be performed.

Regarding the use of titanium grommets, which are intended to reduce fracture rates, some authors claim that grommets improve longevity [14, 31]. In contrast, other authors claim they do not [23]. Furthermore, titanium wear debris from

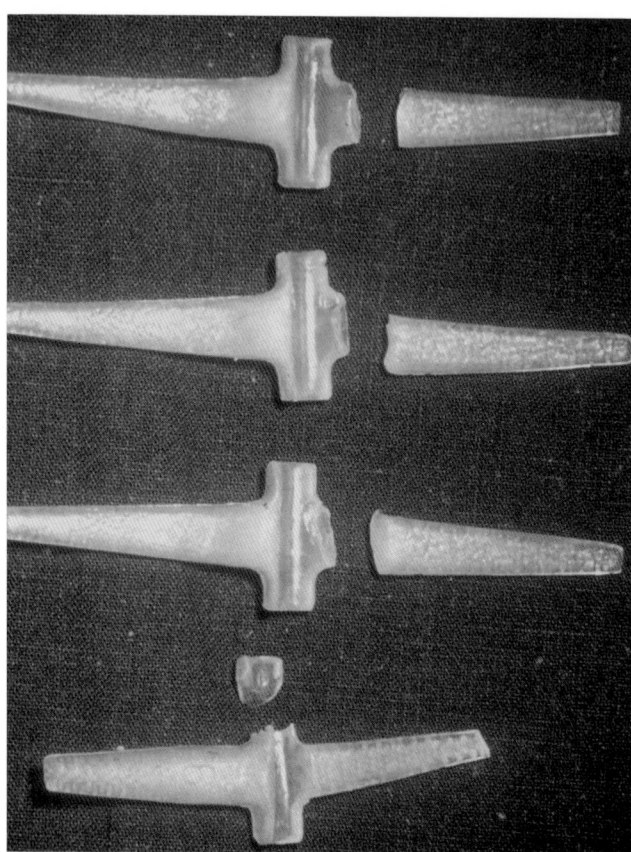

Fig.5.2 *Ex vivo* Swanson metacarpophalangeal prostheses taken from the hand of one patient, from index finger at *top* to little finger at *bottom*

Swanson wrist and thumb implants has been reported [32], though, as with the debate on silicone synovitis, these joints are likely to be more heavily loaded than the metacarpophalangeal joint.

In engineering terms, fatigue is defined as the progressive, localised, and permanent structural damage that occurs when a material is subjected to cyclic or fluctuating strains at nominal stresses that have maximum values less than (often much less than) the static yield strength of the material. Fatigue is recognised as an important cause of engineering failures.

It is recognised that implant fracture is important when single-piece silicone metacarpophalangeal prostheses are considered [33]. If the number of fractures could be reduced, it might be expected that prostheses would function as intended for longer and thus benefit patients for a greater duration. Before cases of fracture can be reduced, the origins of fracture need to be understood, so that the appropriate corrective solutions can be applied.

5.2
Analysis of Explanted Sutter Metacarpophalangeal Prostheses

5.2.1
Clinical Details

With such a failure analysis in mind, 12 Sutter metacarpophalangeal prostheses were obtained from the hands of three patients, who were aged 56–66 years at surgery [15]. Two patients were women, one was a man. All suffered from rheumatoid arthritis. Two of the hands were dominant. The prostheses were retrieved at a mean of 42 months after implantation. The largest prosthesis was a size 50, the smallest a size 10, nine were size 30 or 40. There were 11 fractures, 10 of which were total, so that the initial single-piece implant was now in two pieces.

5.2.2
Macroscopic Analysis

All of the ten total fractures occurred at the junction of the distal stem and the hinge of the Sutter metacarpophalangeal prosthesis. Figure 5.3 shows the explants taken from the hand of patient 2. As can be seen, three of the explants had fractured completely. The fourth explant, which was removed from the patient's index finger, had almost completely fractured. Only a small sliver of material remained to join the palmar aspect of the distal stem with the hinge. This piece of evidence indicated that fracture was initiated on the dorsal aspect of the distal stem and travelled in a palmar direction.

Figure 5.4 shows a side elevation of the two parts of one of the fractured Sutter metacarpophalangeal prostheses from patient 3. The central hinge region has been denoted, as has the distal stem and its dorsal aspect. On the latter, the crack has been initiated before travelling in a palmar direction.

Given that the initiation of fracture has been identified on the dorsal aspect of the distal stems, what additional information can be gained from the fracture faces? Figure 5.5 gives a view of the hinge region, showing the fracture face of an implant from patient 2. What needs to be pointed out is the rectangular shape of the fracture face. This profile matches almost exactly that of the distal stem, and indicates that stresses were highest where the stem and hinge met. These stresses could have been reduced if larger radii were used at these junctions on the implant. This is one example of how the design could be improved and valuable information can be learnt from explants.

5.2.3
Microscopic Analysis

Following a macroscopic visual examination, the fractured prostheses were then sliced so that, after washing and gold-coating, the two fracture faces of each prosthesis could be examined using a Hitachi S-4700 scanning electron microscope. The scanning electron

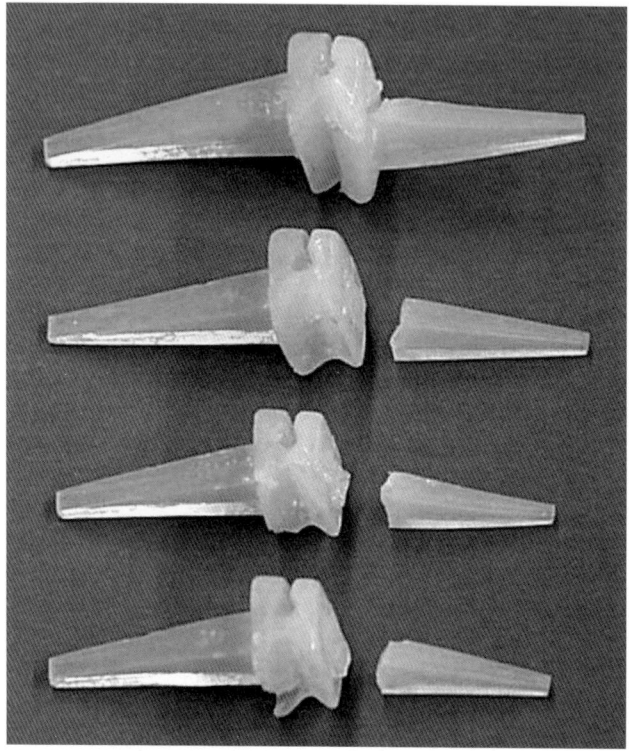

Fig. 5.3 *Ex vivo* Sutter metacarpophalangeal prostheses taken from the hand of one patient, from index finger at top to little finger at bottom

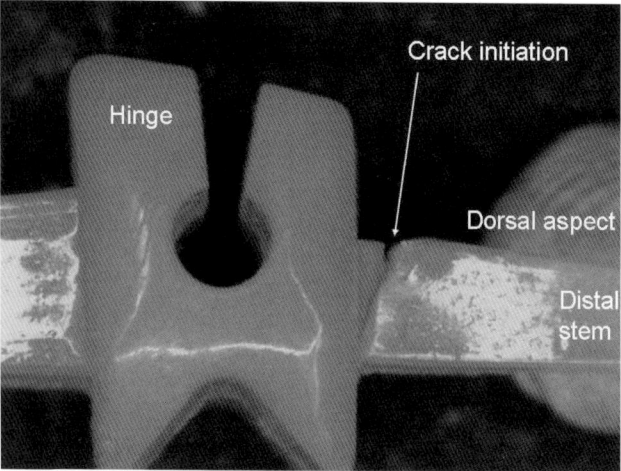

Fig. 5.4 Central section of *ex vivo* Sutter metacarpophalangeal prosthesis, side elevation

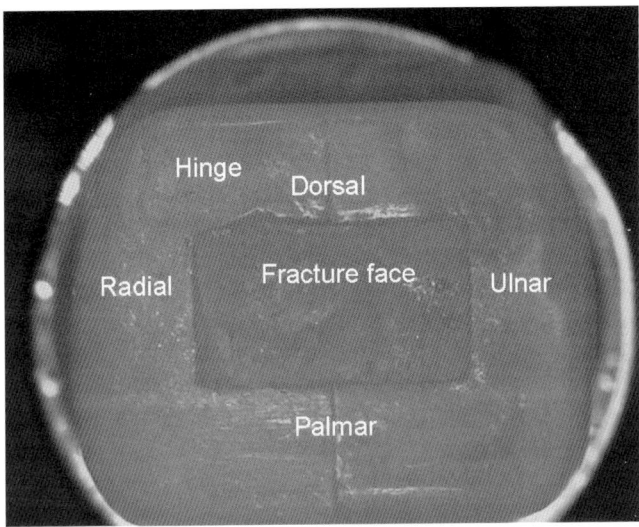

Fig. 5.5 View of fracture face and hinge section of explanted Sutter metacarpophalangeal prosthesis

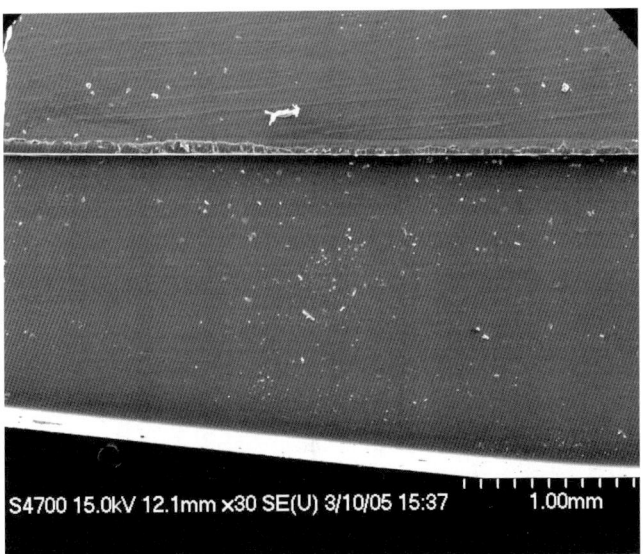

S4700 15.0kV 12.1mm ×30 SE(U) 3/10/05 15:37   1.00mm

Fig. 5.6 Dorsal aspect of new stem of Sutter metacarpophalangeal prosthesis

microscope is pre-eminent in the study of fracture surfaces [34]. In total, 158 scanning electron microscope images were obtained and studied.

Before studying the fracture faces themselves, Figure 5.6 shows the dorsal aspect of the distal stem of a new Sutter metacarpophalangeal prosthesis. The surface is uniform except for the moulding line running horizontally along its length.

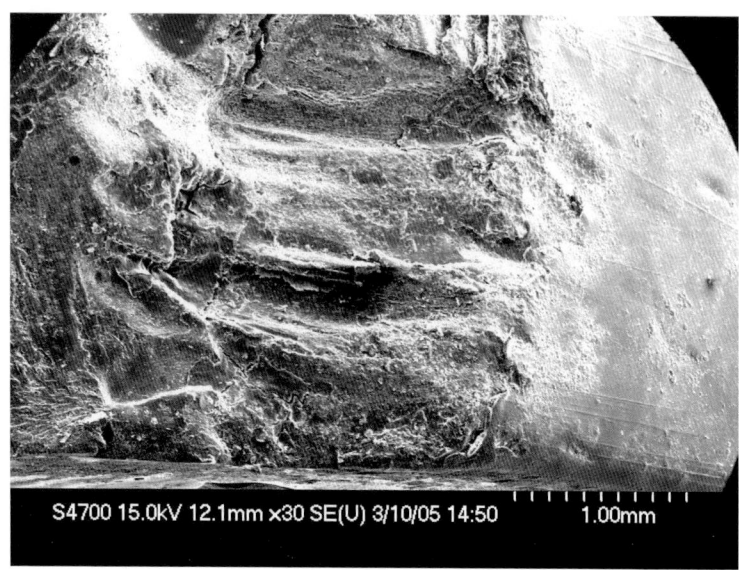

S4700 15.0kV 12.1mm ×30 SE(U) 3/10/05 14:50   1.00mm

Fig. 5.7 Abrasion of dorsal aspect of distal stem of *ex vivo* Sutter metacarpophalangeal prosthesis

In contrast, Figure 5.7 shows the dorsal aspect of a distal stem from an explant, slightly distal to the fracture face. Figures 5.6 and 5.7 are at the same magnification, therefore it can be seen that substantial damage occurred to the dorsal aspect of the distal stem of the prosthesis *in vivo*. As indicated in Figure 5.7, silicone material appears to have been gouged away from the stem when the implant was in the body. This was likely to have been caused by bone impingement from the cortical bone of the proximal phalanx, due to the subluxing forces which dominate in rheumatoid metacarpophalangeal joints. There was relatively little damage on the palmar aspect of the stem.

Fractography is the science of the study of fracture faces. Figure 5.8 shows the radial aspect of the proximal fracture face from the prosthesis fitted in the little finger of patient 1. The dorsal, palmar and radial aspects are indicated. What can also be seen are what are known as 'radial marks' [35]. On fractured surfaces they help to indicate the origin of fracture which, just as Figures. 5.4 and 5.7 have indicated, is on the dorsal aspect. Some areas of abrasion on the dorsal aspect of the stem can also be seen.

Staying with the same fracture face but moving in an ulnar direction takes us to Figure 5.9. Again, dorsal, palmar, radial and ulnar aspects are indicated. So too are the 'radial marks'. These have been additionally indicated by the straight white lines. What can also be seen from this figure is a characteristic feature of fatigue topography known as 'beach marks' [35]. To aid understanding, typical beach marks have been indicated by the dotted white lines. Beach marks are so named as they look like the contours left by waves on a beach. These marks indicate the direction of crack propagation, which is perpendicular to the beach marks. These beach marks therefore allow the direction of crack propagation to be followed, as shown by the dark arrows. What can also be seen is another 'classic' feature of fatigue fracture, the 'shear lip', which indicates the final area of fracture [35].

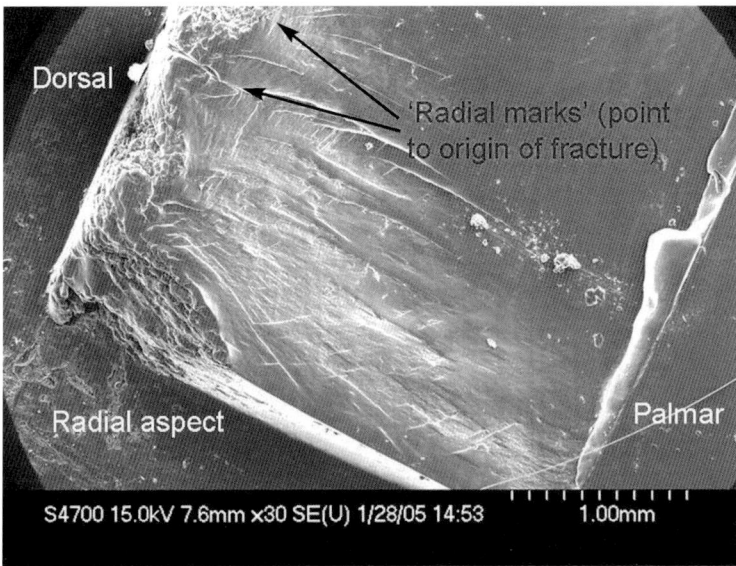

Fig. 5.8 Radial aspect of proximal fracture face of *ex vivo* Sutter metacarpophalangeal prosthesis taken from little finger of patient 1

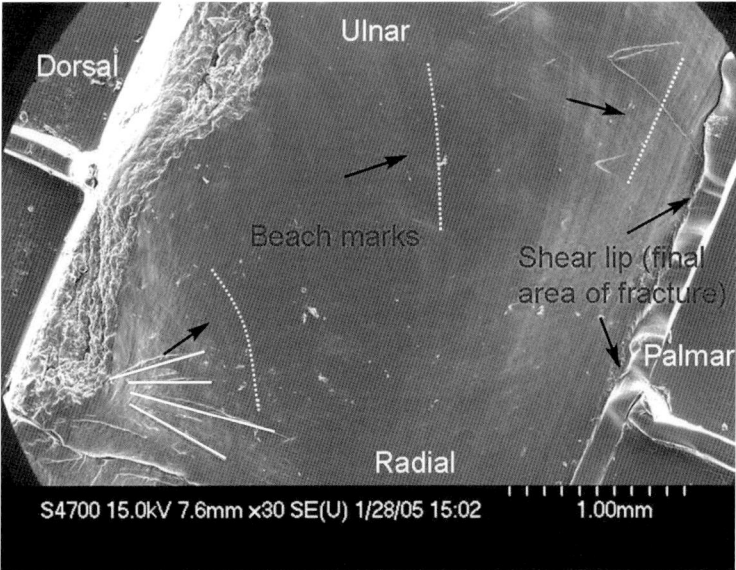

Fig. 5.9 Medial aspect of proximal fracture face of *ex vivo* Sutter metacarpophalangeal prosthesis taken from little finger of patient 1

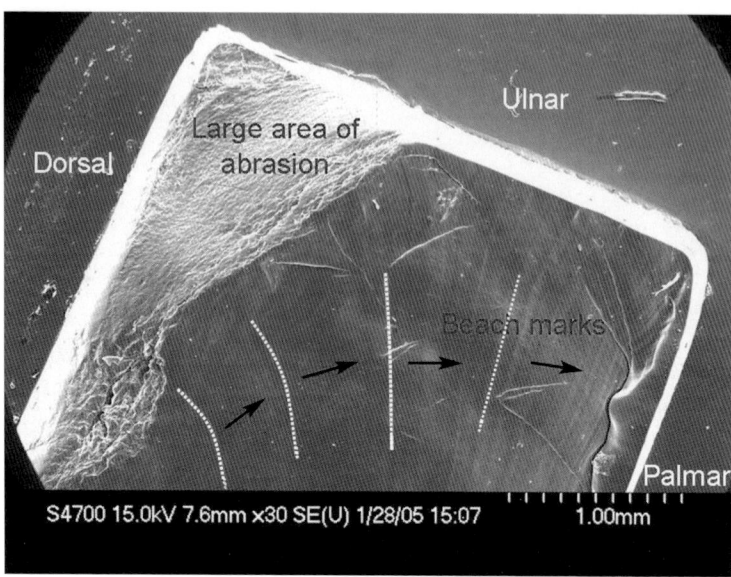

Fig. 5.10 Ulnar aspect of proximal fracture face of *ex vivo* Sutter metacarpophalangeal prosthesis taken from little finger of patient 1

Figure 5.10 shows the ulnar aspect of the same fracture face; again the beach marks can be discerned. Once more these have been indicated by the dotted white lines, and the direction of crack propagation is shown by the arrows. What is also clear from the image is the large area of abrasion damage on the dorsal aspect, likely to be caused by bone impingement. However, while a relatively large amount of silicone material has been removed from the distal stem, this removal has not directly led to fracture of the implant.

The findings from the fracture face of the failed flexible prosthesis removed from the little finger of patient 1 can now be summarised. Abrasion damage is seen on the dorsal aspect of the distal stem of the prosthesis. The 'radial marks' indicate the origin of fracture on the dorsal aspect, towards the radial side. The 'beach marks' show fatigue crack propagation in an arc. The 'shear lip' on the palmar aspect indicates the final area of fracture. Therefore it can be summarised that the crack direction was from radial to ulnar and from dorsal to palmar.

Given this body of evidence, fracture can be explained in the following way. Initially, small cuts are produced by sharp spurs from the finger bones. It is also important to note that Swanson and Sutter prostheses flex at the stem rather than the hinge [36], which means that flexing *in vivo* is occurring at an unintended point. Rheumatoid arthritis causes subluxing forces to dominate in the metacarpophalangeal joints. In turn this means that the cortical bone of the proximal phalanx impinges on the dorsal aspect of the distal stem of the prosthesis. Over time, the crack grows and fatigue failure occurs. While this theory has been postulated previously, it is argued that these images offer the first proof of this hypothesis.

However, there are still unanswered questions. Figure 5.11 shows the distal fracture face of the failed prosthesis taken from the little finger of patient 3. As can be seen,

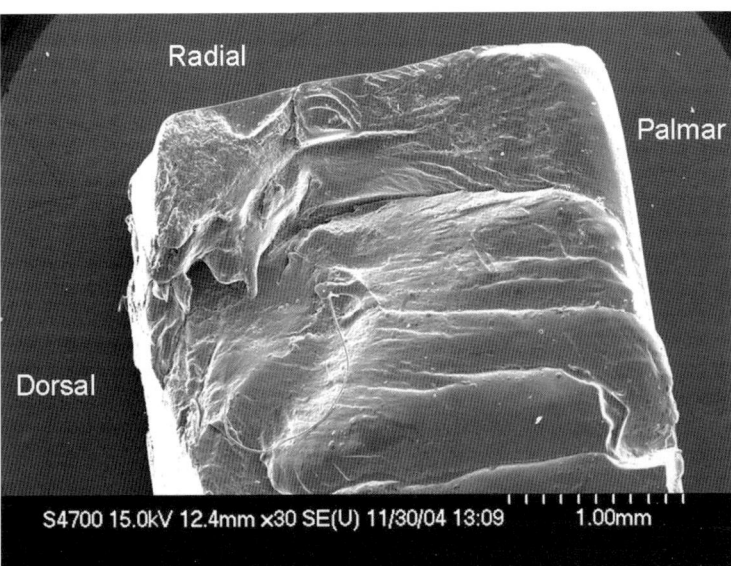

Fig. 5.11 Ulnar aspect of proximal fracture face of *ex vivo* Sutter metacarpophalangeal prosthesis taken from little finger of patient 3

none of the 'classic' fatigue fracture features – radial marks, beach marks, a shear lip – can be seen here. So although fracture was still at the junction of the distal stem and hinge of the prosthesis, it may be that a different form of fracture had occurred. A number of possible explanations can be offered. It is likely there are inevitable differences between patients and between fingers, which will influence fracture faces. In addition it is possible that a single event, such as a blow or a heavy impact, could cause fracture. Thirdly, and perhaps most importantly, fracture faces can be damaged in the period after fracture and pre-removal, which could remove evidence of fatigue failure.

5.3
Looking Ahead

Given the evidence offered in this chapter, it is worth asking how flexible metacarpophalangeal joint prostheses can be improved. Firstly, as has been shown, valuable information can be learnt from explants so such studies should be carried out. Secondly, appropriate *in vitro* testing can be undertaken, rather than new designs of implant, or changes to designs, being tested in human subjects [37]. It should also be appreciated that new biomaterials are being developed all the time. These include improvements to the silicones that are used in flexible implants, as well as other 'conventional' biomaterials such as cobalt chrome, titanium and polyethylene, all of which could be used as materials for finger prostheses. The results offered in this chapter show the value of the concept of the titanium grommets offered with the Swanson prosthesis. However, as some hand surgeons prefer not to fit the grommets, perhaps some method of locally strengthening the material on the dorsal aspect of the stem may have value.

Improved finger prosthesis designs could also be produced: anatomical designs, those which more closely match the shape of the natural metacarpophalangeal joint, could offer a solution, but they generally demand earlier surgical intervention – which patients are naturally less inclined to accept – and when later intervention occurs, results have generally been disappointing [6]. Perhaps the opportunity exists for biomaterials informed and inspired by natural materials, possibly based on the concepts of tissue engineering, to replace our currently available, homogeneous biomaterials. Some useful work related to metacarpophalangeal prostheses has already been done in this area [38, 39]. Equally, it should be appreciated that in the 21st century, significant numbers of failures of new designs of finger prosthesis continue to occur [40–42]. Therefore, despite the best efforts of bioengineers and hand surgeons over several decades, the need for improved metacarpophalangeal prostheses remains.

Acknowledgements
Mr. Rick Milner, consultant plastic surgeon at the Royal Victoria Infirmary in Newcastle upon Tyne in the UK kindly supplied the explanted Sutter prostheses which formed the basis of this chapter.

Summary

❯ Single-piece silicone flexible prostheses dominate the metacarpophalangeal implant market. Most that fail do so by fracture at the junction of the distal stem and the hinge. The main cause of this fracture is rheumatoid arthritis and the loading that this produces at the diseased metacarpophalangeal joints. Usually, a crack is initiated on the dorsal aspect of the distal stem, close to the hinge, and propagated by fatigue, leading to failure of the implant.

References

1. Symmons D, Turner G, Webb R, Asten P et al (2002) The prevalence of rheumatoid arthritis in the United Kingdom: new estimates for a new century. Rheumatology 41:793–800.
2. Ghattas L, Mascella F, Pomponio G (2005) Hand surgery in rheumatoid arthritis: state of the art and suggestions for research. Rheumatology 44:834–845.
3. Chung KC, Kotsis SV, Kim HM et al (2006) Reasons why rheumatoid arthritis patients seek surgical treatment for hand deformities. Journal of Hand Surgery 31:289–294.
4. Combe B (2007) Early rheumatoid arthritis: strategies for prevention and management. Best Practice and Research Clinical Rheumatology 21:27–42.
5. Norwegian Arthroplasty Register, Nasjonalt Register for Leddproteser, http://www.haukeland.no/nrl/eng/Rapport2008.pdf (accessed 4 December 2008).
6. Joyce TJ (2004) Currently available metacarpophalangeal prostheses: their designs and

prospective considerations. Expert Review of Medical Devices 1:193–204.

7. Swanson AB (1972) Flexible implant arthroplasty for arthritic finger joints. Journal of Bone and Joint Surgery (American Volume) 54A:435–456.

8. Joyce TJ, Unsworth A (2002) A literature review of 'failures' of the Swanson finger prosthesis in the metacarpophalangeal joint. Hand Surgery 7:139–146.

9. Wilson YG, Sykes PJ, Niranjan NS (1993) Long-term follow up of Swanson's silastic arthroplasty of the metacarpophalangeal joints in rheumatoid arthritis. Journal of Hand Surgery 18B:81–91.

10. Hansraj KK, Ashworth CR, Ebramzadeh E et al (1997) Swanson metacarpophalangeal joint arthroplasty in patients with rheumatoid arthritis. Clinical Orthopaedics and Related Research 342:11–15.

11. Chung KC, Kowalski CP, Kim HM, Kazmers IS (2000) Patient outcomes following Swanson silastic metacarpophalangeal joint arthroplasty in the rheumatoid hand: a systemic overview. Journal of Rheumatology 27:1395–1402.

12. Chung KC, Kotsis SV, Kim HM (2004) A prospective outcomes study of Swanson metacarpophalangeal joint arthroplasty for the rheumatoid hand. Journal of Hand Surgery 29:646–653.

13. Linscheid RL (2000) Implant arthroplasty of the hand: retrospective and prospective considerations. Journal of Hand Surgery (American Volume) 25A:796–816.

14. Swanson AB, de Groot Swanson G, Ishikawa H (1997) Use of grommets for flexible resection arthroplasty of the metacarpophalangeal joint. Clinical Orthopaedics and Related Research 342:22–33.

15. Joyce TJ, Milner RH, Unsworth A (2003) A comparison of ex vivo and in vitro Sutter metacarpophalangeal prostheses. Journal of Hand Surgery 28B:86–91.

16. Bass RL, Stern PJ, Nairus JG (1996) High implant fracture incidence with Sutter silicone metacarpophalangeal arthroplasty. Journal of Hand Surgery 21A:813–818.

17. McArthur PA, Milner RH (1998) A prospective comparison of Sutter and Swanson silastic spacers. Journal of Hand Surgery 23B:574–577.

18. Parkkila T, Belt EA, Hakala M et al (2005) Comparison of Swanson and Sutter metacarpophalangeal arthroplasties in patients with rheumatoid arthritis: a prospective and randomized trial. Journal of Hand Surgery 30:1276–1281.

19. Moller K, Sollerman C, Geijer M et al (2005) Avanta versus Swanson silicone implants in the MCP joint – a prospective, randomized comparison of 30 patients followed for 2 years. Journal of Hand Surgery 30B:8–13.

20. Delaney R, Trail IA, Nuttall D (2005) A comparative study of outcome between the Neuflex and Swanson metacarpophalangeal joint replacements. Journal of Hand Surgery: Journal of the British Society for Surgery of the Hand 30:3–7.

21. Joyce TJ, Unsworth A (2005) NeuFlex metacarpophalangeal prostheses tested in vitro. Journal of Engineering in Medicine 219:105–110.

22. Synnott K, Mullett H, Faull H, Kelly EP (2000) Outcome measures following metacarpophalangeal joint replacement. Journal of Hand Surgery 25B:601–603.

23. Trail I, Martin J, Nuttall D, Stanley J (2004) Seventeen-year survivorship analysis of silastic metacarpophalangeal joint replacement. Journal of Bone and Joint Surgery 86B:1002–1006.

24. Goldfarb CA, Stern PJ (2003) Metacarpophalangeal joint arthroplasty in rheumatoid arthritis. Journal of Bone and Joint Surgery 85A:1869–1878.

25. Kay AG, Ljeffs JV, Scott JT (1978) Experience with silastic prostheses in the rheumatoid hand: a five year follow up. Annals of the Rheumatic Diseases 37:255–258.

26. Gellman H, Stetson W, Brumfield RH et al (1997) Silastic metacarpophalangeal joint arthroplasty in patients with rheumatoid arthritis. Clinical Orthopaedics and Related Research 342:16–21.

27. Jensen CM, Boeckstyns MEH, Kristiansen B (1986) Silastic arthroplasty in rheumatoid metacarpophalangeal joints. Acta Orthopaedica Scandinavica 57:138–140.

28. Weightman B, Simon S, Rose R et al (1972) Environmental fatigue testing of silastic finger

joint prostheses. Journal of Biomedical Material Research Symposium 3:15–24.

29. Hilker A, Miehlke RK, Schmidt K (2007) Endoprothetik des Fingergrundgelenks. Zeitschrift für Rheumatologie 66:366–375.

30. Bieber EJ, Weiland AJ, Volenec-Dowling S (1986) Silicone rubber implant arthroplasty of the metacarpophalangeal joints for rheumatoid arthritis. Journal of Bone and Joint Surgery Am 68A:206–209.

31. Schmidt K, Willburger RE, Ossowski A, Miehlke RK (1999) The effect of the additional use of grommets in silicone implant arthroplasty of the metacarpophalangeal joints. Journal of Hand Surgery 24B:561–564.

32. Khoo CTK, Davison JA, and Ali M, (2004) Tissue reaction to titanium debris following Swanson arthroplasty in the hand: a report of two cases. Journal of Hand Surgery: Journal of the British Society for Surgery of the Hand 29:152–154.

33. Weiss A-PC, Moore DC, Infantolino C et al (2004) Metacarpophalangeal joint mechanics after 3 different silicone arthroplasties. Journal of Hand Surgery 29:796–803.

34. Bhowmick AK, De SK (eds) (1991) Fractography of rubbery materials, Elsevier Applied Science, London.

35. Parrington RJ (2002) Fractography of metals and plastics. Practical Failure Analysis 2:16–19 and 44–46.

36. Gillespie TE, Flatt AE, Youm Y, Sprague BL (1979) Biomechanical evaluation of metacarpophalangeal joint prosthesis designs. Journal of Hand Surgery 4A:508–521.

37. Joyce TJ (2003) Personal view. Snapping the fingers. Journal of Hand Surgery 26B:566–567.

38. Honkanen PB, Kellomaki M, Lehtimaki MY et al (2003) Bioreconstructive joint scaffold implant arthroplasty in metacarpophalangeal joints: short-term results of a new treatment concept in rheumatoid arthritis patients. Tissue Engineering 9:957–965.

39. Waris E, Ashammakhi N, Lehtimaki M et al (2008) Long-term bone tissue reaction to polyethylene oxide/polybutylene terephthalate copolymer (Polyactive(R)) in metacarpophalangeal joint reconstruction. Biomaterials 29:2509–2515.

40. Radmer S, Andresen R, Sparmann M (2003) Poor experience with a hinged endoprosthesis (WEKO) for the metacarpophalangeal joints. Acta Orthopaedica Scandinavica 74:586–590.

41. Field J, (2008) Two to five year follow-up of the LPM ceramic coated proximal interphalangeal joint arthroplasty. Journal of Hand Surgery, European Volume 33:38–44.

42. Hobby JL, Edwards S, Field J, Giddins G (2008) A report on the early failure of the LPM Proximal Interphalangeal Joint Replacement. Journal of Hand Surgery, European Volume 33:526–527.

Abstract Rheumatoid arthritis is a chronic systemic auto-immune inflammatory disease which may affect all parts of the body but predominantly afflicts the limb joints. Despite progress in medical therapy, a high number of patients still face the destructive and deforming sequelae of the disease, in part because of a late, inadequate, or refused early pharmacological treatment. Flexible prostheses, like the Swanson, rely on the elastic properties of their material for their performance. Surface replacement prostheses are partially able to reproduce the physiological sliding of the bony segments but require the capsulo-ligamentous structure of the joint to be in a suitably good condition. Hinged prostheses rely on their coupling mechanism to provide stability in a given range of motion, but inherent weakness of the recipient bone and incompleteness of the capsulo-ligamentous structures may cause their failure. Flexible prostheses are the option but, strictly speaking, they cannot be defined as true prosthetic devices because their design does not enable the restoration of an adequate range of motion and strength.

Keywords Hinged Prostheses • Metacarpophalangeal Joint • Pathophysiology • Rheumatoid Arthritis • Spacers • Surface Replacement Prostheses

6.1
Introduction

Rheumatoid arthritis (RA) is a chronic systemic auto-immune inflammatory disease which may affect all parts of the body but predominantly afflicts the limb joints. Women are affected more commonly than men.

The pathology shows a chronic erosive synovitis affecting the synovial membrane around the joints and tendons. The progress of the synovitis may be described in three stages: first synovial involvement, in which permanent histological or functional damage are not detectable; secondly cartilaginous damage, in which the inflamed synovial membrane infiltrates the cartilaginous tissue (Fig. 6.1) – this may lead to joint instability with tendon rupture and joint and tendon dislocation; and thirdly development of a massive fibrosis which causes stiffness of the joint and structural deformity.

F. Catalano (✉)
Orthopaedics and Hand Surgery, The Catholic University School of Medicine, Rome, Italy

A. Merolli, T.J. Joyce (eds), *Biomaterials in Hand Surgery.*
© Springer-Verlag Italia 2009

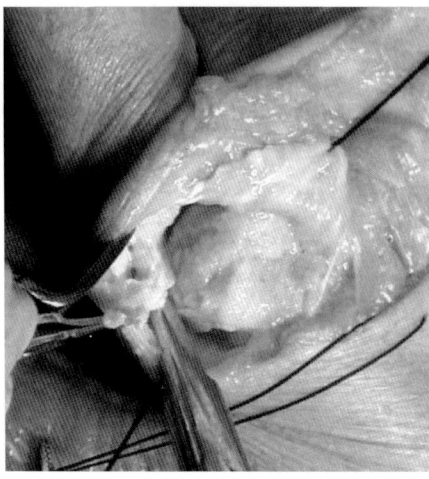

Fig. 6.1 A chronic erosive synovitis affecting the synovial membrane around the joints and tendons produced this cartilaginous damage on the dorsal aspect of the second metacarpal head

RA is, unfortunately, quite common. About ten years from the onset, half of patients develop significant joint alterations that may severely impair activities in everyday life and even force them to abandon employment; even life expectancy is reduced by rheumatoid arthritis.

The efficacy of drug therapy has recently been boosted by the so-called "biological response modifiers". It is known that some cytokines sustain the chronic inflammatory state that characterizes RA, so specific drugs have been developed aimed at counteracting these cytokines by three main mechanisms: being soluble receptors for the cytokines; being monoclonal antibodies against the cytokines; and being antagonists for the cytokine receptors.

However, despite progress in medical therapy, a high number of patients still face the destructive and deforming sequelae of the disease, in part because of late, inadequate, or refused early pharmacological treatment.

Deformity and functional impairment arise because of gradual progressive destruction of the capsulo-ligamentous structures and degeneration of the joint surfaces. The fingers drift in an ulnar direction and are partially dislocated volarly at the level of the metacarpophalangeal (MCP) joint. Proximal and distal interphalangeal joints (PIP and DIP joints) may be affected to various degrees.

6.2
Prosthetic Surgical Treatment

In cases where pain and functional impairment have progressed too far, two surgical options may be proposed: joint fusion or prosthetic replacement.

Prostheses can be grouped into three main categories: joint spacers; surface replacement prostheses; and hinged prostheses.

Joint spacers, which allow a minimal range of motion and restore some distance between the bony segments, rely on the elastic properties of their material for their performance.

Surface replacement prostheses are partially able to reproduce the physiological sliding of the bony segments, in terms of both geometry and range of motion, but require the capsulo-ligamentous structure of the joint to be in a suitably good condition.

Hinged prostheses rely completely on their coupling mechanism to provide stability in a given range of motion.

Several designs, in all three categories, may be employed to replace a PIP or DIP joint in a rheumatoid patient, but for the MCP joint replacements the most practiced option is the polymeric flexible spacer, such as the Swanson design. Surface replacement in rheumatoid arthritis would require the competence of a surgically restored capsulo-ligamentous structure and this is often not possible at the advanced stage of disease already reached by many of the patients who require surgery. Hinged prostheses, after some time *in vivo*, have tended to show breakage in the hinge or loosening at the bone–stem interface.

6.3
Pathological Physiology

The wrist, carpus, and digital rays have to be considered as a single kinematic chain and, for this reason, deformities produced in any proximal joint may affect and worsen more distal joints.

The wrist is often considered the prime mover in the sequential appearance of deformities in the hand. Radiocarpal instability favors diminished competence of the volar ligamentous structures, prompting partial volar dislocation of the carpus. The latter condition, and the associated instability of the distal radio-ulnar joint, contributes to the eventual rupture of the overstretched extensor tendons.

The partial volar dislocation of the carpus impairs the balance between flexor and extensor tendons and this will, in turn, produce a hyperextension of the MCP joints and flexion of the PIP joints, a deformity known as "boutonnière" (button-hole).

When the capsular-ligamentous structures at the MCP joints are destroyed, the fingers are dislocated in volar and ulnar directions, carrying the extensor tendons along and making them intrude into the intermetacarpal space, so producing the typical ulnar drift deformity of the rheumatoid hand (Fig. 6.2).

A reduction in grip strength is associated with diminished length between the insertions of the flexor muscles, which is produced by the partial volar dislocation of the carpus.

6.3.1
Involvement of the Wrist

About 75% of patients presenting the late stages of RA show significant deformity at the wrist. Early onset may start from the ulnar, central, or radial side but ulnar onset is the most common.

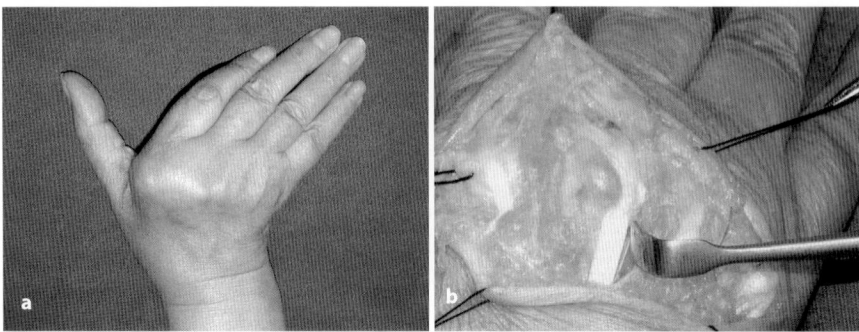

Fig. 6.2 Fingers drift in an ulnar direction (**a**) and are partially dislocated volarly at the level of the metacarpophalangeal joint, carrying the extensor tendons along and making them intrude into the intermetacarpal space (**b**)

6.3.1.1
Ulnar Onset

In ulnar onset, the diminished competence of the radial-ulnar-carpal ligaments favors partial volar dislocation of the carpus and dorsal dislocation of the ulnar head, which jointly impair the pronation and supination at the wrist. Volar dislocation of the extensor carpi ulnaris transforms this extensor muscle into an actual flexor, further worsening volar dislocation and ulnar deviation of the carpus and stretching the lunate attachments. When the radial-carpal ligaments are spared, they maintain the navicular bone firmly in place but, in so doing, there is an ulnarward stretch of the proximal carpal row, coupled with a radial stretch of the more distal structures (distal carpal row and metacarpal bones) and this worsens the ulnar drift of the hand. The eventual irregular surfaces produced in the dorsal carpus by this deformity can be a factor in promoting rupture of the extensor tendons. In the so-called "caput ulnae syndrome", rupture of the tendon of the extensor digiti minimi is the first to appear, giving the picture of the "blessing hand", while rupture of the other extensors may follow in an ulnar-radial sequence.

6.3.1.2
Central Onset

When central onset is encountered, the radio-navicular-ulnar ligaments are affected first; this may be due to a relatively rich vascularization. Rupture of the lunonavicular interosseous ligament may soon follow-with the eventual ulnarward deviation of the lunate and the proximal sinking of the capitate towards the radial articular cartilage; the latter occurrence will later evolve into a global decrease in carpal height. Intrinsic muscles gain a mechanical advantage by these changes, setting the basis for the "swan neck" deformity of the fingers.

6.3.1.3
Radial Onset

A radial onset is quite rare. The radio-navicular-capitate ligament is affected first and the deformity will later evolve into a decreased carpal height with a volar dislocation and a predominant attitude in pronation.

Without surgical treatment, wrist deformity in RA may lead to three main conditions: a distal radio-ulnar instability with a variable degree in functional limitation of the pronation-supination; a fibrotic stiffness among the carpal bones which, while having a positive influence in reducing pain, strongly favors more distal deformities of the fingers; and severe damage at the level of the ligamentous structures of the carpus, which is characterized by intense pain, volar dislocation, and rupture of both the flexor and extensor tendons (well described as a "carpal collapse").

6.3.2
Involvement of the Metacarpophalangeal Joints

The metacarpophalangeal joints are affected in about half of rheumatoid patients. As a consequence there is: volar-ulnar dislocation of the extensor tendons; ulnar deviation of the fingers; and partial volar dislocation of the proximal phalanges (Fig. 6.3).

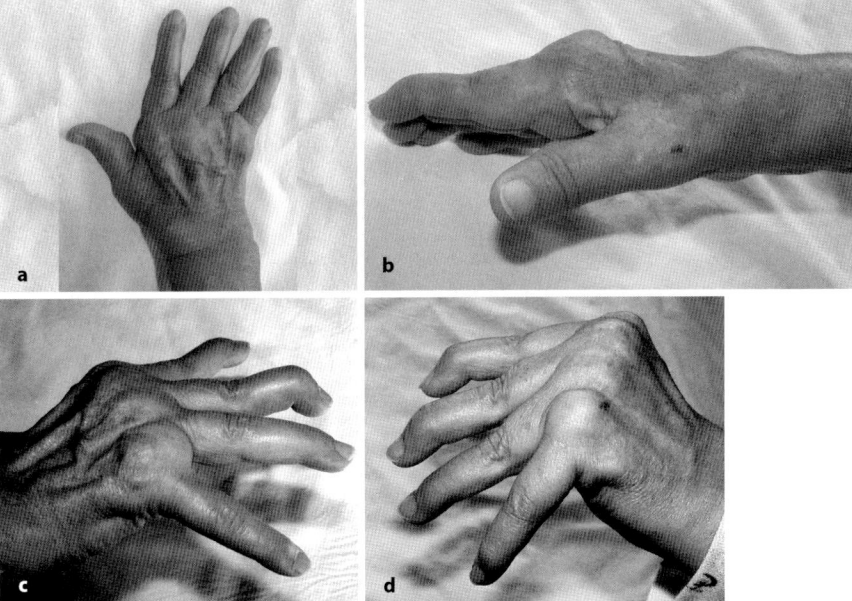

Fig. 6.3 A patient presenting the ulnar drift of the fingers and a Z-thumb deformity (**a**). The wrist is often considered the prime mover in the sequential appearance of deformities in the hand; radiocarpal instability favors diminished competence of the volar ligamentous structures, prompting partial volar dislocation of the carpus (**b**).The index and middle fingers show a swan neck deformity (**c**). The proximal phalanges are partially dislocated volarly (**d**)

In the MCP joint the bone segments are stabilized by several structures, including the lateral bands; these are asymmetric constraints since those on the ulnar side are thicker and tougher. Rupture of the weaker radial band is a first stage in the development of the ulnar drift of the hand, coupled with the ulnarward traction cumulatively exerted by the muscles (only on the 4th finger are the muscular actions quite balanced in all planes). On the volarly, partially dislocated fingers, the advantageous action of the extensor tendons on the middle phalanx will produce hyperextension, favoring the development of the swan neck deformity.

6.3.3
Involvement of the Interphalangeal Joints

Deformity at the interphalangeal joints is produced by the imbalance between the flexor and extensor tendons. Hyperextension of the PIP joint coupled with hyperflexion of the DIP characterize the swan neck deformity and this, as already stated, can be the consequence of either a wrist or a MCP joint deformity.

When the dorsal central slip of the extensor tendon is disrupted, the "boutonnière" deformity ensues; this deformity is not the consequence of other more proximal alterations but is produced locally and favors the possible compensatory hyperextension of the DIP and MCP joints.

Synovitis at the DIP joint may be associated with the degenerative rupture of the extensor tendon at its distal insertion at the base of the distal phalanx, leading to the "mallet finger" deformity.

6.4
Problems Associated with Prosthetic Surgery of Metacarpophalangeal Joints in Rheumatoid Patients

Hinged prostheses have been unsuccessful in the prosthetic replacement of MCP joints in rheumatoid patients. Inherent weakness of the recipient bone, leading to periprosthetic fractures, and incompleteness of the capsulo-ligamentous structures were the main causes of early failure of hinged prostheses.

Flexible prostheses, such as the Swanson, are the option in these patients but, strictly speaking, they cannot be defined as true prosthetic devices because their design does not enable the restoration of an adequate range of motion and strength. Swanson's design is basically a spacer which helps to keep the alignment of the digital ray (metacarpal and finger) (Fig. 6.4). Its great flexibility will allow the prosthesis to bend in response to any external force applied to the finger, so care must be taken not to overload the prosthesis even during limited daily activities. However, Swanson's design is effective in relieving pain and improves the cosmetic appearance of the hand; furthermore its long-term follow-up is positive.

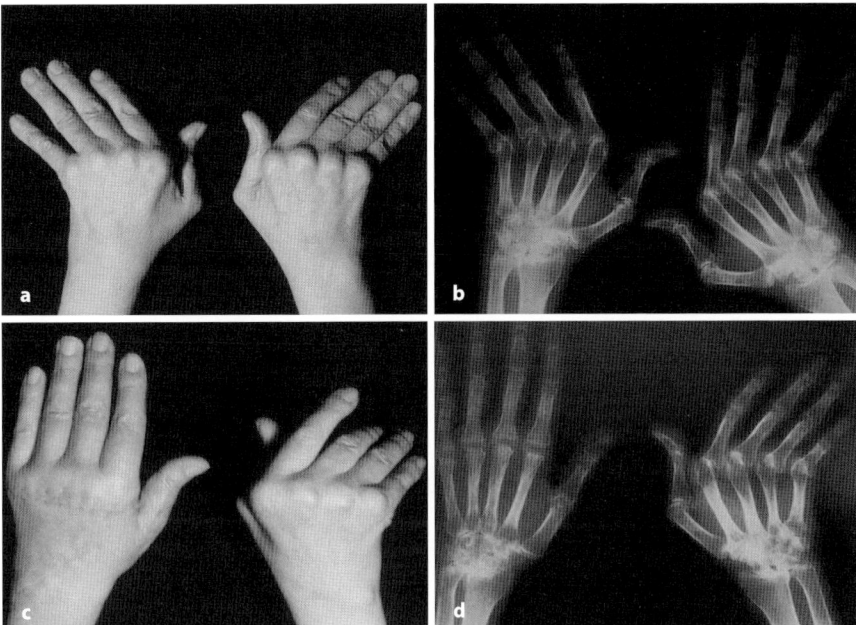

Fig. 6.4 A patient with bilateral involvement (**a**) and the related X-ray appearance (**b**). The left hand received treatment by using the Swanson prosthesis on all the fingers and the fusion of the first metacarpophalangeal joint (**c**). Flexible prostheses help in keeping the alignment of the digital rays (metacarpals and fingers) (**d**). The right hand received the same treatment in a second procedure

The best results may be obtained when only the MCP joints are affected, without the additional involvement of other proximal or distal joints.

The surgical technique may be demanding because the operative field is small and the shafts of the proximal phalanx and the metacarpal bone cannot be moved too far apart to allow introduction of the stems into the bony canals: single-piece designs like the Swanson prosthesis require a significant and totally unphysiological bending during this phase.

The limited operative space and small dimensions should be kept in mind while modeling any new MCP joint prosthesis.

Bone stock availability may be variable from patient to patient and there are cases where erosion has depleted a significant amount of the bone shaft. Osteoporosis may be present in those patients who have a long history of limited use of the hands because of pain, but it may also be caused by long-term treatment with corticosteroids. These drugs are also responsible for severe damage to the capsulo-ligamentous structures.

Swanson's "prosthesis", despite its limitations, can be considered the best option available, when long-term clinical results are considered. Similar flexible polymeric prostheses have been developed following its principles.

However, the intrinsic stability of the Swanson prosthesis is very limited and a kind of fibrotic encapsulation must be achieved to help in preventing the recurrence of ulnar drift and volar dislocation of the proximal phalanxes, among all the other deformities. Accessory surgical steps may be of prime importance, followed by a prolonged dynamic (during the day) and static (during the night) splinting.

Accurate planning of all the steps that the individual patient may require is very important; some patients do need preliminary correction at the level of more proximal joints before commencing treatment at the MCP joint. An ulnar deviation of the carpus, with a dorsal dislocation of the ulnar head and possible rupture of the extensor tendons, needs to be treated in advance, otherwise a MCP joint prosthesis, despite being correctly implanted, will follow the same fate as the natural joint and the patient will end up with a prosthetized ulnar-drifted hand, in about a couple of weeks (Fig. 6.5).

A dynamic splint which stresses towards the radial side may be ineffective if the carpus is not recentered; this repositioning must be achieved before proceeding to implant prostheses in the MCP joints.

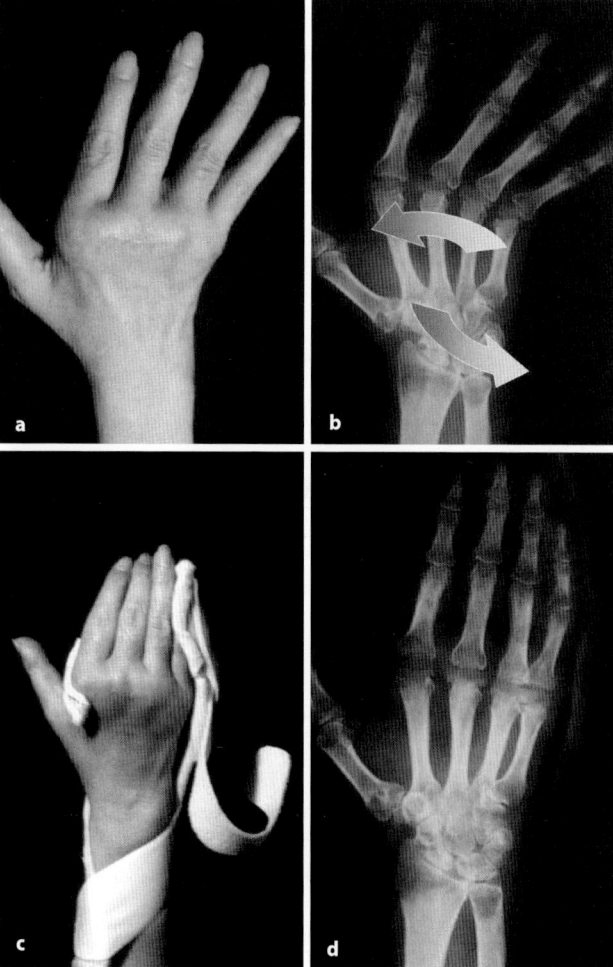

Fig. 6.5 Accurate planning of all the steps is very important; some patients do need preliminary correction at the level of more proximal joints, otherwise MCP joint prostheses, despite being correctly implanted, will follow the same fate as the natural joint and the patient will end up with a prosthetized ulnar-drifted hand (**a**); this repositioning (opposite to the *arrows*) must be achieved before proceeding to implant prostheses in the MCP joints (**b**), and its effectiveness may be demonstrated by a splint (**c**, **d**)

The carpus in the rheumatoid patient leans in an ulnar direction and then tends to supinate. After splinting, a radio-navicular-ulnar fusion, or, more simply, a radionavicular fusion, may suffice in its stabilization.

If a "Z thumb" ensues following the rupture of the extensor pollicis brevis tendon, fusion of the first MCP joint to correct the "Z thumb" deformity should be performed before undertaking any prosthetic surgery of the MCP joints of the fingers.

Swan neck deformity of the interphalangeal joints must be corrected before implanting MCP prostheses.

The hypercontraction of the interossei muscles promotes flexion at the MCP joints; if this effect is moderate, it will be enough to dissect the lumbricals and interossei tendons by a dorsal approach to obtain a volar release; flexor tendon mobilization may also be obtained by the same dorsal approach. However, in cases of severe flexion contracture, the lumbricals and interossei tendons require a volar approach to be effectively released.

Retraction of the abductor digiti minimi is often significant and needs release. Collateral ligaments of the second and third finger, even if preserved, may be lengthened and weakened, so they need to be reinforced by suturing.

Finally, it is most important to recenter the volar-ulnar dislocated extensor tendons on the dorsum of the new MCP joint.

Early mobilization requires splinting. In the author's opinion, custom-made dynamic splints are the most effective. Dynamic splints promote the advantageous active movements but prevent those that may favor recurrence of the deformity. Ulnar drift is always likely to recur, so splinting may be required for several months. Passive splinting must be installed during the night.

Infections following MCP joint prostheses are rare.

Prosthetic fractures are not infrequent but, fortunately, fracture of a flexible prosthesis does not lead to discomfort in those cases where an effective encapsulation was achieved. A fractured flexible prosthesis, which has been well encapsulated, may still allow flexion–extension at the MCP joint.

Silicone synovitis, despite being greatly feared, is seldom encountered.

Further Reading

Abboud JA, Beredjiklian PK, Bozentka DJ (2003) Metacarpophalangeal joint arthroplasty in rheumatoid arthritis. J Am Acad Orthop Surg 11:184–191.

Al-Ahaideb A, Drosdowech DS, Pichora DR (2006) Fractional flexor tendon lengthening for advanced metacarpophalangeal flexion contracture in rheumatoid hands. J Hand Surg [Am] 31:1690–1693.

Alderman AK, Ubel PA, Kim HM et al (2003) Surgical management of the rheumatoid hand: consensus and controversy among rheumatologists and hand surgeons. J Rheumatol 30:1464–1472.

Beevers DJ, Seedhom BB (1995) Design of a non-constrained, non-cemented, modular, metacarpophalangeal prosthesis. Proc Inst Mech Eng [H] 209:185–195.

Beevers DJ, Seedhom BB (1995) Metacarpophalangeal joint prostheses. A review of the clinical results of past and current designs. J Hand Surg [Br] 20:125–136.

Bielefeld T, Neumann DA (2005) The unstable metacarpophalangeal joint in rheumatoid arthritis: anatomy, pathomechanics, and physical rehabilitation considerations. J Orthop Sports Phys Ther 35:502–520.

Bogoch ER, Escott BG, Judd MG (2008) Insufficient flexion of the metacarpophalangeal joint of the little finger following Swanson silicone arthroplasty for rheumatoid arthritis. Hand (NY) 3:24–29.

Boyer MI, Gelberman RH (1999) Operative correction of swan-neck and boutonnière deformities in the rheumatoid hand. J Am Acad Orthop Surg 7:92–100.

Burezq H, Polyhronopoulos GN, Beaulieu S et al (2005) The value of radial collateral ligament reconstruction and abductor digiti minimi release in metacarpophalangeal joint arthroplasty. Ann Plast Surg 54:397–401.

Burgess SD, Kono M, Stern PJ (2007) Results of revision metacarpophalangeal joint surgery in rheumatoid patients following previous silicone arthroplasty. J Hand Surg [Am] 32:1506–1512.

Burr N, Pratt AL, Smith PJ (2002) An alternative splinting and rehabilitation protocol for metacarpophalangeal joint arthroplasty in patients with rheumatoid arthritis. J Hand Ther 15:41–47.

Chacko AT, Rozental TD (2008) The rheumatoid thumb. Hand Clin 24:307–314, vii.

Chinchalkar SJ, Pitts S (2006) Dynamic assist splinting for attenuated sagittal bands in the rheumatoid hand. Tech Hand Up Extrem Surg 10:206–211.

Chung KC, Kotsis SV, Kim HM et al (2006) Reasons why rheumatoid arthritis patients seek surgical treatment for hand deformities. J Hand Surg [Am] 31:289–294.

Clark DI, Delaney R, Stilwell JH et al (2001) The value of crossed intrinsic transfer after metacarpophalangeal silastic arthroplasty: a comparative study. J Hand Surg [Br] 26:565–567.

Day CS, Ramirez MA (2006) Thumb metacarpophalangeal arthritis: arthroplasty or fusion? Hand Clin 22:211–220.

De Santolo A, Briceño L, De Santolo G, Cevedo N (2008) Stabilization of finger ulnar deviation in rheumatoid arthritis: extensor indicis proprius tenodesis. J Hand Surg [Am] 33:450–453.

Delaney R, Trail IA, Nuttall D (2005) A comparative study of outcome between the Neuflex and Swanson metacarpophalangeal joint replacements. J Hand Surg [Br] 30:3–7.

Dell PC, Renfree KJ, Below Dell R (2001) Surgical correction of extensor tendon subluxation and ulnar drift in the rheumatoid hand: long-term results. J Hand Surg [Br] 26:560–564.

DiBenedetto MR, Lubbers LM, Coleman CR (1991) Relationship between radial inclination angle and ulnar deviation of the fingers. J Hand Surg [Am] 16:36–39.

Fowler NK, Nicol AC (2001) Functional and biomechanical assessment of the normal and rheumatoid hand. Clin Biomech (Bristol, Avon) 16:660–666.

Fowler NK, Nicol AC (2001) Long-term measurement of metacarpophalangeal joint motion in the normal and rheumatoid hand. Proc Inst Mech Eng [H] 215:549–553.

Fowler NK, Nicol AC (2002) A biomechanical analysis of the rheumatoid index finger after joint arthroplasty. Clin Biomech (Bristol, Avon) 17:400–405.

Gnjidić Z, Kurtagić N (1990) Relationship between finger and wrist deformities in rheumatoid arthritis. Acta Med Iugosl 44:233–241.

Goldfarb CA, Dovan TT (2006) Rheumatoid arthritis: silicone metacarpophalangeal joint arthroplasty indications, technique, and outcomes. Hand Clin 22:177–182.

Goldfarb CA, Stern PJ (2003) Metacarpophalangeal joint arthroplasty in rheumatoid arthritis. A long-term assessment. J Bone Joint Surg Am 85A(10):1869–1878.

Gossec L, Baro-Riba J, Bozonnat MC et al (20050) Influence of sex on disease severity in patients with rheumatoid arthritis. J Rheumatol 32:1448–1451.

Harris D, Dias JJ (2003) Five-year results of a new total replacement prosthesis for the finger metacarpo-phalangeal joints. J Hand Surg [Br] 28:432–438.

Herren DB, Simmen BR (2002) Shortening osteotomy for treatment of metacarpophalangeal joint deformity. Clin Orthop Relat Res 394:186–191.

Honkanen PB, Kellomäki M, Lehtimäki MY et al (2003) Bioreconstructive joint scaffold implant arthroplasty in metacarpophalangeal joints: short-term results of a new treatment concept in rheumatoid arthritis patients. Tissue Eng 9:957–965.

Ikävalko M, Skyttä ET, Belt EA (2007) One-year results of use of poly-L/D-lactic acid joint scaffolds and bone packing in revision metacarpophalangeal arthroplasty. J Hand Surg Eur Vol 32:427–433.

Ito J, Koshino T, Okamoto R, Saito T (2003) Radiologic evaluation of the rheumatoid hand after synovectomy and extensor carpi radialis longus transfer to extensor carpi ulnaris. J Hand Surg [Am] 28:585 590.

Joyce TJ, Milner RH, Unsworth A (2003) A comparison of ex vivo and in vitro Sutter metacarpophalangeal prostheses. J Hand Surg [Br] 28:86–91.

Kimball HL, Terrono AL, Feldon P, Zelouf DS (2003) Metacarpophalangeal joint arthroplasty in rheumatoid arthritis. Instr Course Lect 52:163–174.

Kleinert HE, Sunil TM (2005) Use of volar plate for reconstructing the radial collateral ligament after metacarpophalangeal arthroplasty of fingers in rheumatoid arthritis: surgical technique. J Hand Surg [Am] 30:390–393.

Linscheid RL (2000) Implant arthroplasty of the hand: retrospective and prospective considerations. J Hand Surg [Am] 25:796–816.

Mandl LA, Burke FD, Shaw Wilgis EF et al (2008) Could preoperative preferences and expectations influence surgical decision making? Rheumatoid arthritis patients contemplating metacarpophalangeal joint arthroplasty. Plast Reconstr Surg 121:175–180.

Mandl LA, Galvin DH, Bosch JP et al (2002) Metacarpophalangeal arthroplasty in rheumatoid arthritis: what determines satisfaction with surgery? J Rheumatol 29:2488–2491.

Massy-Westropp N, Johnston RV, Hill C (2008) Post-operative therapy for metacarpophalangeal arthroplasty. Cochrane Database Syst Rev 1:CD003522.

Massy-Westropp N, Krishnan J (2003) Postoperative therapy after metacarpophalangeal arthroplasty. J Hand Ther 16:311–314.

Möller K, Sollerman C, Geijer M et al (2005) Avanta versus Swanson silicone implants in the MCP joint – a prospective, randomized comparison of 30 patients followed for 2 years. J Hand Surg [Br] 30:8–13.

Parker WL, Rizzo M, Moran SL et al (2007) Preliminary results of nonconstrained pyrolytic carbon arthroplasty for metacarpophalangeal joint arthritis. J Hand Surg [Am] 32:1496–1505.

Parkkila T, Belt EA, Hakala M et al (2005) Comparison of Swanson and Sutter metacarpophalangeal arthroplasties in patients with rheumatoid arthritis: a prospective and randomized trial. J Hand Surg [Am] 30:1276–1281.

Parkkila T, Hakala M, Kautiainen H et al (2006) Osteolysis after Sutter metacarpophalangeal arthroplasty: a prospective study of 282 implants followed up for 5.7 years. Scand J Plast Reconstr Surg Hand Surg 40:297–301.

Parkkila TJ, Belt EA, Hakala M et al (2006) Survival and complications are similar after Swanson and Sutter implant replacement of metacarpophalangeal joints in patients with rheumatoid arthritis. Scand J Plast Reconstr Surg Hand Surg 40:49–53.

Pereira JA, Belcher HJ (2001) A comparison of metacarpophalangeal joint silastic arthroplasty with or without crossed intrinsic transfer. J Hand Surg [Br] 26:229–234.

Pettersson K, Wagnsjö P, Hulin E (2006) NeuFlex compared with Sutter prostheses: a blind, prospective, randomised comparison of Silastic metacarpophalangeal joint prostheses. Scand J Plast Reconstr Surg Hand Surg 40:284–290.

Rozental TD (2007) Reconstruction of the rheumatoid thumb. J Am Acad Orthop Surg 15:118–125.

Silva PG, Lombardi I Jr, Breitschwerdt C et al (2008) Functional thumb orthosis for type I and II boutonniere deformity on the dominant hand in patients with rheumatoid arthritis: a randomized controlled study. Clin Rehabil 22:684–689.

Sunil TM, Kleinert HE (2006) Fashioning a new radial collateral ligament during arthroplasty of the finger metacarpophalangeal joints in rheumatoid arthritis. Tech Hand Up Extrem Surg 10:79–86.

Taylor TH, Eranki KP, Kerin KD (2007) Intrinsic muscle spasm of the hand; Bunnell's sign. J Rheumatol 34:1332–1335.

Thomsen NO, Boeckstyns ME, Leth-Espensen P (2003) Value of dynamic splinting after replacement of the metacarpophalangeal joint in patients with rheumatoid arthritis. Scand J Plast Reconstr Surg Hand Surg 37:113–116.

Trail IA, Martin JA, Nuttall D, Stanley JK (2004) Seventeen-year survivorship analysis of silastic metacarpophalangeal joint replacement. J Bone Joint Surg Br 86:1002–1006.

Watson HK, Weinzweig J, Guidera PM (1997) Sagittal band reconstruction. J Hand Surg [Am] 22:452–456.

Williamson SC, Feldon P (1995) Extensor tendon ruptures in rheumatoid arthritis. Hand Clin 11:449–459.

Wilson RL, Carlblom ER (1989) The rheumatoid metacarpophalangeal joint. Hand Clin 5:223–237.

Requirements for a Metacarpophalangeal Joint Prosthesis for Rheumatoid Patients and Suggestions for Design

7

A. Merolli

Abstract Requirements for a metacarpophalangeal joint prosthesis for rheumatoid patients are defined and suggestions for a new design are described. The reason for designing such a prosthesis is to propose a better solution for the most required indication of a metacarpophalangeal joint artificial replacement. The most important clinical requirement is the ability to perform a task even in the absence of any significant capsulo-ligamentous structure, because it is likely that most patients will require the arthroplasty in a late stage of the disease. A self-stable prosthetic articulation and circular cross-sectional stems are suggested; the latter may bring an advantage in improved transfer of stresses at the stem–bone interface. To cope with the requirement of a self-stable design, allowing limited but long-lasting load bearing, a limitation in the range of motion of the implant is suggested.

Keywords Biomaterials • Computer-assisted Design • Metacarpophalangeal Joint • Rheumatoid Arthritis

7.1
Introduction

Why design a metacarpophalangeal (MCP) joint prosthesis exclusively for the rheumatoid patient?

An appropriate answer may be that when designing a prosthesis for the MCP joint, the goal is to solve problems associated with its most required indication, namely rheumatoid arthritis (RA). The dedicated design of a MCP prosthesis that is solely applicable in the RA patient can be a rewarding accomplishment, even at the price of the limitations that such a prosthesis may bring in terms of range of motion, or the limitation that such a dedicated prosthesis may be less suitable for other, less common, needs such as joint replacement following trauma or degenerative arthrosis.

A. Merolli (✉)
Orthopaedics and Hand Surgery, The Catholic University School of Medicine, Rome, Italy

A. Merolli, T.J. Joyce (eds), *Biomaterials in Hand Surgery.*
© Springer-Verlag Italia 2009

95

7.2
Four-dimensional Kinematics of the Metacarpophalangeal Joint

Biomechanical modeling of the MCP joint kinematics may be the starting point for designing a MCP joint prosthesis for the RA patient [1].

It is known that a two-dimensional (2D) plot describes the relationship between two variables (x,y); the way to produce and interpret this kind of plot is well established. A 3D plot describes the relationship between three variables (x,y,z). A 2D plot can be defined as a 3D plot in which one of the three variables has a constant value.

Three-dimensional plots were arduous to produce before the advent and widespread distribution of microcomputers and this limited their use and the consequent knowledge yielded from their interpretation.

The kinematics of the MCP joint of the index finger in the human hand have been analyzed in the past by a computerized opto-electronic system [2, 3]; the three Eulerian angles of flexion–extension, abduction–adduction, and axial rotation as a function of time were measured (Fig. 7.1). Plotting these three angular parameters versus time gave three 2D plots which were compared together to investigate a possible standard pattern of motion. However, comparison of the three different 2D plots was not able to provide an intuitive description of the pattern of motion.

It was noticed that by imposing the experimental condition of having a continually increasing value in one parameter (namely flexion), a 3D plot could be used to describe effectively the relationship between the four variables measured (1, flexion–extension; 2, abduction–adduction; 3, axial rotation; and 4, time). Graphical software devoted to this task was produced, and analysis of "3D/4-variable plots" of a series of experimental measurements was undertaken. The movement analyzed was the flexion of the index finger starting from an hyperextended position with respect to the metacarpus, which was kept fixed by a suitably shaped holder. Optical markers were fixed to the finger.

The subjects were asked to perform the movement in two modalities: fast or slow. The three Eulerian angles were measured as a function of time, with a positive progression of numerical values from extension to flexion, from adduction to abduction, and from pronation to supination (from now on, flexion–extension will be referred to as "flexion"; abduction–adduction as "deviation"; and pronation–supination as "rotation").

Since the values of flexion always increase, the reading of time can be linked to that of flexion itself. In detail, the constant time interval between two values (which was the sampling interval of 0.01 s) can be visualized by two 3D peaks so that the magnitude of time is given by the density of peaks along the direction of flexion.

The peaks of each tetrad of values (1, flexion–extension; 2, abduction–adduction; 3, axial rotation; and 4, time) are connected by a line, and a simple computer animation produces their sequential blinking, giving a highly effective perception of variation in flexion angular velocity during movement.

Although the subjects were asked to perform in only two modalities (fast or slow movements), analysis revealed the existence of three classes of movements, namely: 1, rapid movements; 2, intermediate movements; and 3, slow movements. The duration of rapid movements was up to 0.15 s. Intermediate movements lasted between 0.16 s and

0.41 s. Slow movements were recorded from 0.48 s to 1.76 s. A simple and repetitive representation of each class of movement can be derived (a canonical form).

In the canonical form of a rapid movement (Fig. 7.1d), rotation values are high at the beginning, then decrease in the middle and, finally, increase again. A concentration of peaks (3–5) was present at the start (slow start), then there was a bell-shaped profile of flexion angular velocity without any agglomeration of peaks at the end of the movement (no significant "brake" before the end). A certain degree of coupling can be described

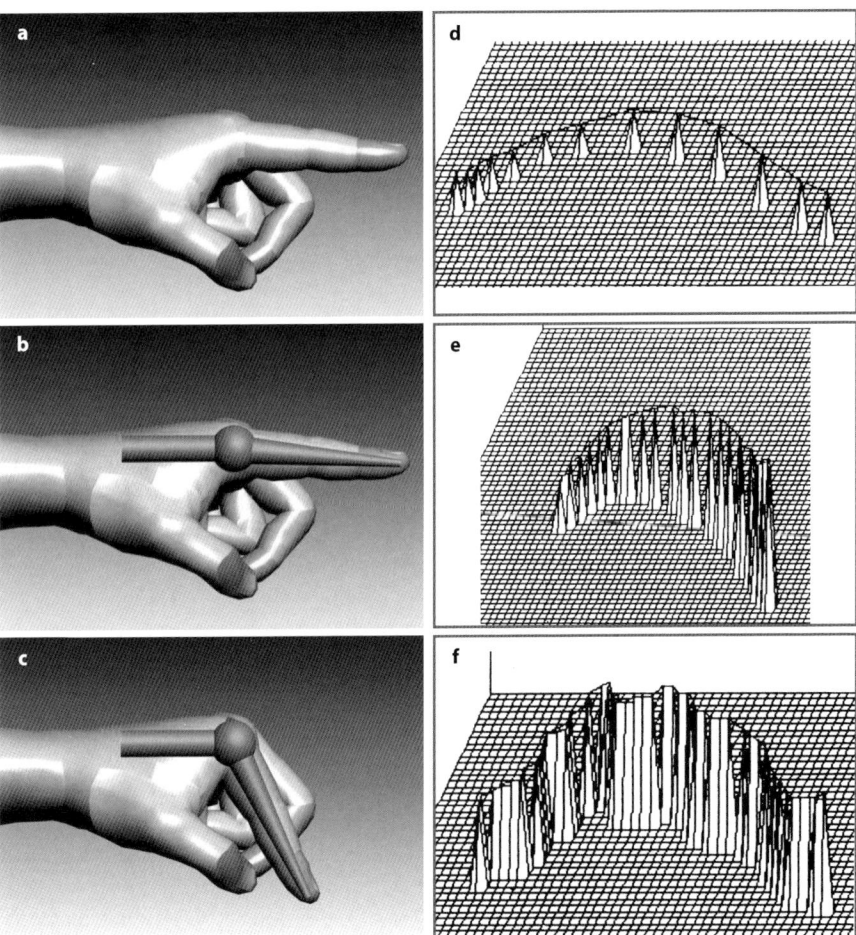

Fig. 7.1 The kinematics of the metacarpophalangeal joint of the index finger have been analyzed by a computerized opto-electronic system; the movement analyzed was flexion of the index finger (**a-c**). In the canonical form of a rapid movement (**d**), rotation values are high at the beginning, then decrease in the middle and, finally, increase again; the profile of flexion angular velocity is bell shaped. The intermediate movement (**e**) maintains basically the same profile, while the slow movement (**f**) is characterized by gross variations in the rate of increase of angular velocity. It seems as if slow movements are generated by a superimposition of several rapid movements. The x axis corresponds to flexion; the y axis to deviation and the z axis to rotation

between deviation and rotation: in detail, at the inversion in sign of rotational values there is a slow-down (flexure point) in the rate of increase of deviation velocity.

The canonical form of an intermediate movement (Fig. 7.1e) maintains basically the same profile for rotational values, which are high at the beginning, decrease in the middle, and then increase again. It is, however, difficult to discern the presence of the other characteristics ascribed to rapid movements.

The canonical form of a slow movement (Fig. 7.1f) is typically characterized by gross variations in the rate of growth of angular velocity; this peculiarity is quite well visualized by the computer animation which shows how flexion angular velocity "starts and stops" two, three, or more times during the movement. It seems as if slow movements are generated by a superimposition of several rapid movements.

From these observations it can be inferred that the rapid movement plot describes the pattern of motion that is basically due to the mechanical constraints of the joint. In intermediate and, more so, in slow movements, the pattern of motion reveals the presumed influence of neuromotor control.

7.3
Solid Modeling and Rapid Prototyping

Computer-assisted design (CAD) and computer-assisted manufacture (CAM) have become widely accepted in all fields of engineering during the past 30 years.

More recently, techniques have been proposed for the rapid manufacture of prototypes that assist greatly in manipulating, discussing and modifying a designed object, and enhance understanding between specialists from different fields when they are required to work together on a project (a situation that may arise between orthopedic surgeons and mechanical engineers while discussing a new design for a MCP joint prosthesis).

In principle, the design of an object should not be restricted to the professional "designer" alone, because it is accepted that is often the "final user" who grasps the key points in solving many problems, in terms of both difficulties that must be overcome and the feasibility of possible solutions. In orthopedic surgery, there are several examples of designs that were directly proposed from the outset by orthopedic surgeons.

Among the easiest ways to design a 3D object, the so-called "solid modeling" technique has much to recommend it. With this technique it is possible to design an accurate model of a complex object by the sequential and hierarchical association of simpler geometrical solids, like spheres, cylinders, cubes, etc. Figure 7.2 illustrates how, starting from a few regular solids, a gradual process of fusion and subtraction may generate the graphical model of a proposed MCP joint prosthesis.

Nowadays there are formats for data handling that enable suitable software to generate the appropriate commands for computer-assisted production tools, so that a real object can be manufactured from the solid modeling design alone. However, producing a complex object with materials such as surgically approved metallic alloys may be quite complicated and very costly. Using the technique of rapid prototyping, an object may be produced in polymeric materials in a much less expensive way.

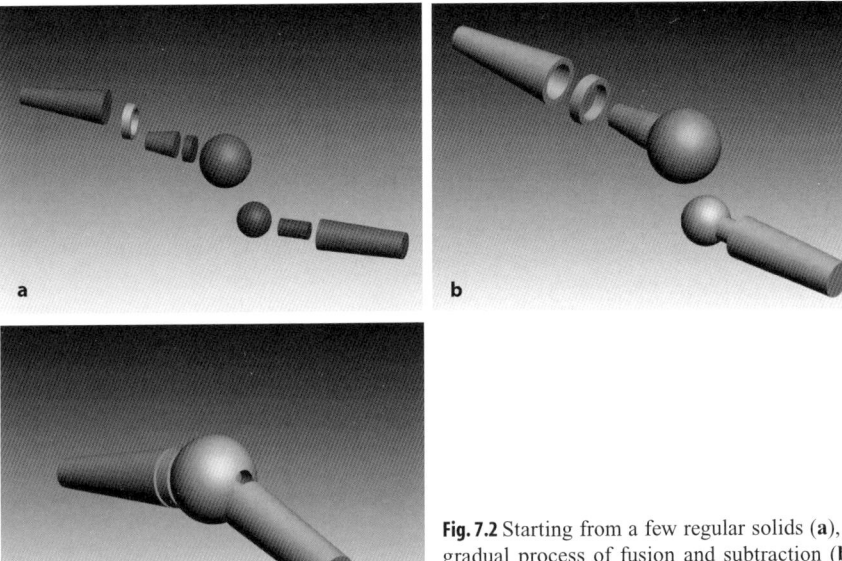

Fig. 7.2 Starting from a few regular solids (**a**), a gradual process of fusion and subtraction (**b**) may generate the graphical model of a proposed MCP joint prosthesis (**c**)

Early rapid-prototyping devices used the holographic photolithography technique, which takes advantage of a laser beam to solidify selected volumes of a viscous polymeric blend. Cheaper and easier devices nowadays use the so-called "three-dimensional plotting" technique; in this way, a 3D object is built up by solidifying a layer of viscous polymeric material slice-by-slice (a process that resembles the 3D graphic reconstructions obtained by computer tomography of a skeletal segment).

Developing new objects using CAD software and rapid-prototyping techniques helps not only in designing the manufacturing process but also in planning the surgical steps eventually needed for implantation of the device. The kinematics of an artificial joint may be tested before actually producing it (Fig. 7.3), so that the design can be modified immediately if it does not comply with a surgical constraint (Fig. 7.4). This may be of particular value in a MCP joint prosthesis, where a significant surgical constraint

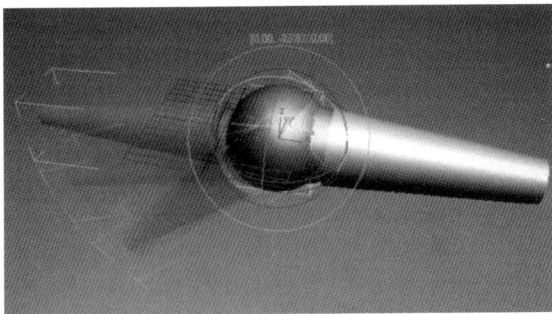

Fig. 7.3 The kinematics of an artificial joint may be tested virtually by CAD, before actually producing it

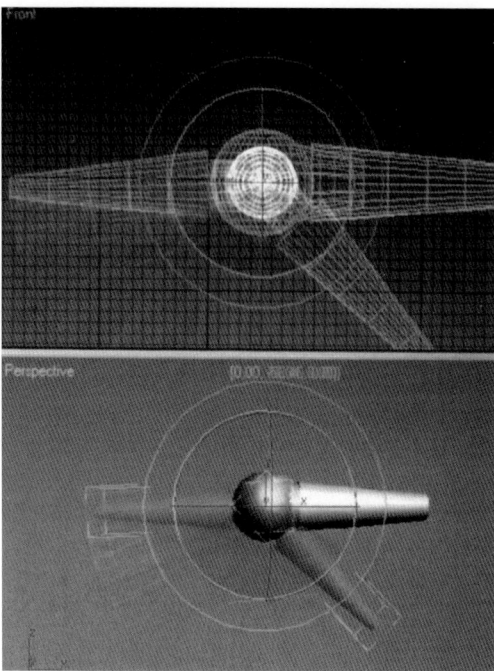

Fig. 7.4 A design can be modified virtually by CAD if it does not comply with a surgical constraint; in this case, the hyperflexion of the joint required for implanting this proposed design would be impossible, as shown by the virtual overlapping of the stems

is the requirement that the two bony segments (the metacarpal bone and the proximal phalanx) cannot be translated too far apart, in an already small surgical field.

7.4
Clinical Requirement

In the author's opinion, the most important clinical requirement for a MCP prosthesis to be used for rheumatoid patients is the ability to perform its task even in the absence of any significant capsulo-ligamentous structure able to keep the joint components in the correct place over the entire range of motion. This is because it is likely that most patients will require the joint arthroplasty in a late stage of the disease, when significant or even complete capsulo-ligamentous degenerative destruction has occurred. This requirement makes several surface-replacement designs unsuitable for the task.

Designs like the Swanson MCP prosthesis proved to be effective in relieving pain and realigning the digital ray [4–8]; these must both be retained by any new design of prosthesis. However, the potential of an increase in load bearing is a new improvement that should be pursued. An adequate achievement would be a long-lasting load-bearing capacity that is useful for daily activities such as combing the hair, holding a glass, or opening a bottle of milk. These actions can be effectively performed with only a fraction of the physiologically available range of motion. Fortunately, the complete range of motion of the MCP joint is not required for most of our activities and this is also the case with the RA patient. A prosthesis that is able to cope with pain, deformity and activities of daily living will probably be well accepted by patients, even if the device does not allow the maximum possible range of physiological flexion and extension.

7.5
Two Surgical Constraints

In the author's experience, there are two main surgical constraints that limit freedom in design, forcing the adoption of solutions with few alternatives.

The first is the need to access the diaphyseal cavities, after the diseased joint has been removed, without pulling the two bony segments (the phalanx and the metacarpal) too far apart; this is normally achieved by hyperflexing the joint. A single-piece flexible prosthesis may be implanted by hyperflexion of its articulation. Hinged designs require different solutions, one is intraoperative assembly of the joint by different kinds of snap-together mechanisms between the proximal and distal stem. In this type of solution the force required for the intraoperative assembly will be the same that, subsequently, the patient could apply, voluntarily or by accident, to disassemble the prosthesis. This is a great limitation for any design that aims to offer the patient load bearing that is suitable for daily life. Another solution is the provision of a joint that is already able to perform the hyperflexion required for its implantation; however, this may be a risk for the patient who could, unwittingly, end up with a prosthesis that is stressed under too much flexion, which in turn could damage the extensor tendon and loosen the proximal stem of the prosthesis. Furthermore, tiny joint components are likely to be required for both solutions and these are prone to break during use.

The second major surgical constraint is the limited space of the operative field; this may be a relevant problem when preparing the bony canals for the stems. It is sometimes difficult to choose the correct sagittal plane of the phalanx prior to reduction and extension of the joint. This constraint, together with the limited and variable availability of bone stock in RA patients, makes it difficult to meet the requirement for highly precise angular alignment of the stems, particularly if their cross-section involves a complex geometry. Stems of circular cross-section (such as cylinders or truncated cones) are, from this point of view, the most appropriate for surgery.

7.6
Choice of Biomaterials

Requirements for the materials to be used in a design with the characteristics proposed in the previous sections, namely a self-stable joint and circular cross-sectional stems, may be demanding. While several different classes of materials have been used in the past for MCP joint prostheses [4], it is likely that only a limited choice will be available to achieve the required performance at a reasonable cost and with accessible technology.

A key requirement should be achievement of the greatest possible reduction in friction and wear in the joint mechanism. This will require the availability of mirror-finished cobalt–chrome metal alloy; however, this must be achieved for components that are far smaller than the ball and socket assembly of hip joint prostheses, for which this technique was refined. In the author's opinion it is not likely that this reduction in friction and wear can be achieved with many other materials. However, technology is progressing rapidly, regarding the manufacturing of micro-artifacts, and the near future could bring other possible solutions.

If metal alloys are used for the articulation, the same materials will be used for the stems, even if the bending and torsional loads on them will be small in magnitude and probably well within the range of mechanical properties of several other classes of non-metallic materials. Having suggested a basically circular cross-section for the stems, a coated interface that is able to guarantee both an immediate and a long-term osteo-integration is necessary. Several options are available in this field: a bioactive ceramic coating would be a good choice.

7.7
A Possible Design

Anatomical and surgical constraints were considered to be of the outmost importance during the design of the MCP joint prosthesis for RA patients (Fig. 7.5a). A weak bone in association with disrupted capsulo-ligamentous structures led to the decision that pre-assembled joint components had to be used to safeguard the mechanical perform-ance of the joint, instead of multiple components which need to be assembled intra-operatively by a snap-in or any other mechanism (Fig. 7.5b).

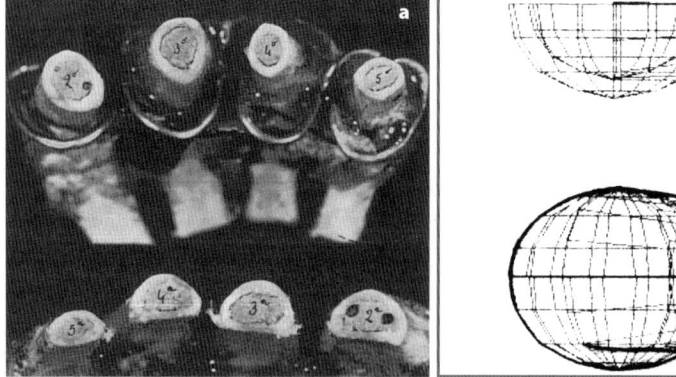

Fig. 7.5 An anatomical preparation which dates back to the 1980s. **a** Cross-section of the metacarpals (*top*) and phalanxes (*bottom*) are anatomical constraints which were studied on cadaveric specimens. **b** A very early design of a hemi-valve (*top*) and of a pre-assembled articu-lation component (*bottom*)

The choice of a pre-assembled joint may be associated with the presence of a single-piece stem coming out from it. If this is the distal stem then implantation will be easier.

As already stated, the limited space of the operative field (Fig. 7.6) and the limited and variable availability of bone stock in RA patients, make it unlikely that highly precise angular alignment of stems with complex geometries can be achieved. Stems of circular cross-section are certainly more "surgical friendly".

Stems of circular cross-section may confer an advantage in transferring stresses at the stem–bone interface. Finite elements have been applied to model implants for the MCP joint [9]. In the present case, a simple finite-element model may be designed in which stems of different cross-sectional shapes fit inside a cylinder that simulates the bone segment (Fig. 7.7). If a torque is applied, stresses are distributed at the interface in a manner that is closely related to the stem's geometry. While high stresses may concen-

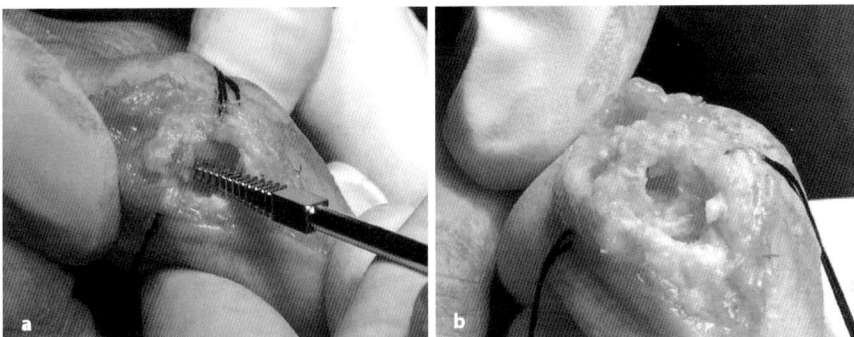

Fig. 7.6 The limited space of the operative field while preparing the canal for the distal stem (**a**) and the limited and variable availability of bone stock in RA patients (**b**) make it unlikely that highly precise angular alignment of stems with complex geometries can be achieved

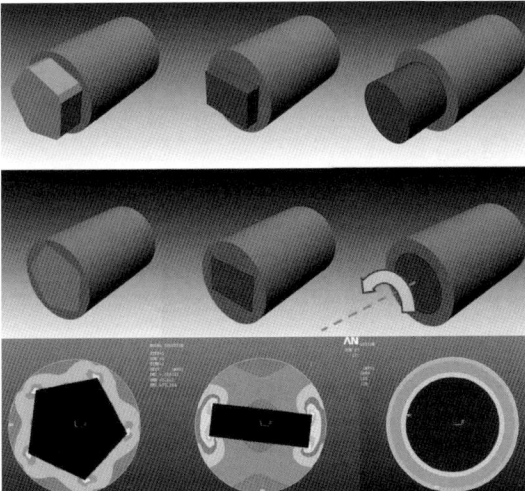

Fig. 7.7 A simple finite-element model may be designed in which stems of different cross-sectional shapes fit inside a cylinder that simulates the bone segment (*top*). If a torque is applied (*middle*), stresses are distributed at the interface in a manner that is closely related to the stem's geometry (*bottom*)

trate where spikes or flanges are present, the most uniform distribution, with the lowest magnitude, is associated with a circular cross-section (as theoretically predicted).

According to the laws of Wolff and Pauwels [10–12], bone rarefaction may occur in areas of non-physiological higher stress, eventually leading to stem loosening and failure of the prosthesis.

A press-fit circular cross-section stem, however, will poorly counteract torsional loads in the early period after implantation. To promote bone apposition and integration, a bioactive-ceramic coating has to be applied (Fig. 7.8). Bone apposition requires time; it is therefore suggested that after implantation of the prosthesis, a period of about three weeks of MCP joint immobilization must be administered; this will bring the advantages of allowing a fibrous-scar tissue to form a new capsule around the joint and allowing time for the bone remodeling process to be established at the bone–coating interface.

A particular feature of the prosthesis, which may be the area of application for future technologies, is the flat groove that accommodates the extensor tendon (Fig. 7.9a).

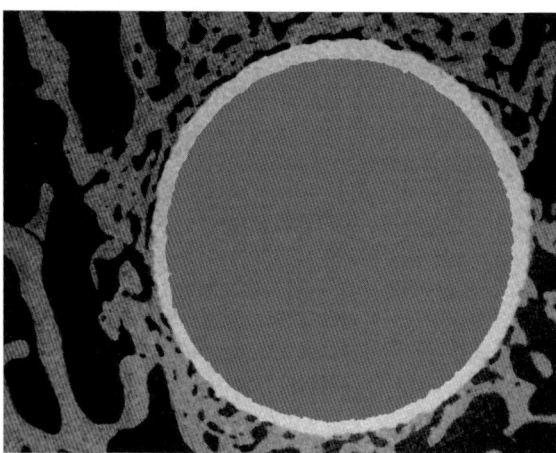

Fig. 7.8 Processed image of a backscattered electron micrograph of a transverse histological section which shows trabecular bone in tight apposition with hydroxyapatite coating (*white*) on a metallic stem (*grey*)

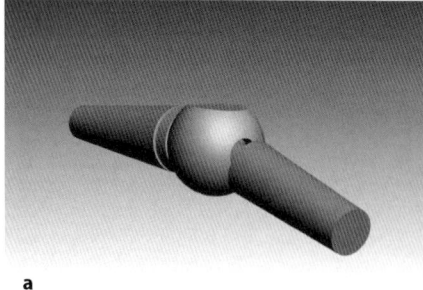

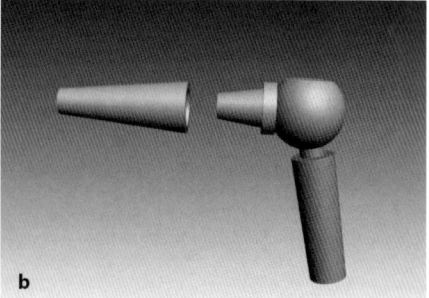

a   b

Fig. 7.9 A particular feature of the prosthesis, which may be the area of application for future technologies, is a flat groove that accommodates the extensor tendon (**a**). Since the pre-assembled stem–articulation complex of the proposed design does not hyperflex, it will be coupled with the proximal stem by a short press-fit cone-morse (**b**), within the space allowed by anatomical constraints

This is envisaged as a mirror-finished metallic component; however, a more sophisticated and partially bioactive coating may be sought, one that could incorporate lubricating molecules implanted in a polymeric layer. Friction between the extensor tendon and the metallic groove could, however, raise some concern regarding the long-term performance when load bearing is applied.

To cope with the strategic clinical requirement of a self-stable design that is able to perform its task even in the absence of any significant capsulo-ligamentous structure, allowing limited but long-lasting load bearing, it is, in the author's opinion, wise to impose a limitation on the range of motion of the implant. The exact values are open to discussion but, in the author's analysis, a range of extension–flexion between –85° and –30° (so, without any actual extension), lateral deviation between +20° and 0° (so, without any actual ulnar deviation) and axial rotation of +10° to –10° would be good in relation to the feasibility of design and effectiveness of clinical performance.

Since the pre-assembled joint does not hyperflex, it will be coupled with the proximal stem by a short press-fit cone-morse (Fig. 7.9b), within the spacing allowed by anatomical constraints.

7.8
Conclusions

Some of the principles and ideas proposed in this chapter can be found in new designs already on the market or in others published in the literature. It is important that research in this field continues and, hopefully, increases, because of its associated high clinical demand.

Acknowledgements
A special thank to Dr. Francesco Mollica and Dr. Maria Silvia Spinelli for the finite-element modeling of Figure 7.7.

References

1. Tamai K, Ryu J, An KN, Linscheid RL et al (1988) Three-dimensional geometric analysis of the metacarpophalangeal joint. J Hand Surg [Am] 13:521–529.
2. Catalano F, Tranquilli Leali P, Fanfani F et al (1980) Metacarpo-phalangeal joint: a biomechanic approach. Acta Orthop Belg 46:678–685.
3. Merolli A, Tranquilli Leali P et al (1994) Three–dimensional four variables plot for the study of metacarpo-phalangeal joint kinematics. In: Schuind F (ed.) Advances in the biomechanics of the hand and wrist. Plenum Publishing, New York, pp 377–382.
4. Beevers DJ, Seedhom BB (1995) Metacarpophalangeal joint prostheses. A review of the clinical results of past and current designs. J Hand Surg [Br] 20:125–136.
5. Rothwell AG, Cragg KJ, O'Neill LB (1997) Hand function following silastic arthroplasty of the metacarpophalangeal joints in the rheumatoid hand. J Hand Surg [Br] 22:90–93.

6. Rittmeister M, Porsch M, Starker M, Kerschbaumer F (1999) Metacarpophalangeal joint arthroplasty in rheumatoid arthritis: results of Swanson implants and digital joint operative arthroplasty. Arch Orthop Trauma Surg 119:190–194.
7. Chung KC, Kowalski CP, Myra Kim H, Kazmers IS (2000) Patient outcomes following Swanson silastic metacarpophalangeal joint arthroplasty in the rheumatoid hand: a systematic overview. J Rheumatol 27:1395–1402.
8. Joyce TJ (2004) Currently available metacarpo–phalangeal prostheses: their design and prospective considerations. Expert Rev Med Device 1:193–204.
9. Penrose JMT, Williams MW, Hose DR, Trowbridge EA (1997) In-situ simulation of one-piece metacarpophalangeal joint implants using finite element analysis. Med Eng Phys 19:303–307.
10. Wolff J (1986) The law of bone remodelling. Springer-Verlag, Berlin Heidelberg.
11. Pauwels F (1976) Developmental effects of the functional adaptation of bone. Anat Anz 139:213–220.
12. Carter DR, Orr TE (1992) Skeletal development and bone functional adaptation. J Bone Miner Res 7(Suppl 2):S389–S395.

Research Trends for Flexor Tendon Repair

8

S. Thomopoulos

Abstract Basic science research on the biology, repair, and rehabilitation of intrasynovial flexor tendon injuries has led to major advances in the clinical management of these injuries. Clinically applicable animal models have been developed to test novel treatments prior to clinical use. Initial research efforts focused on improving the biomechanics of the suture repair and reducing adhesions during healing through passive motion rehabilitation. Recent trends for flexor tendon repair include biological and biomaterial approaches to improve healing. Treatment of the tendon surface with natural and synthetic materials has led to dramatic improvements in the gliding properties of the tendons, and hence the function of the digit. Development of biofactor delivery systems has allowed investigators to test the effects of growth factors for enhanced flexor tendon healing. Application of these new biomaterials to intrasynovial flexor tendon repair has the potential to improve both tendon function (by improving the gliding properties of the tendon) and tendon strength (by enhancing extracellular matrix synthesis).

Keywords Adhesion • Biomaterials • Biomechanics • Delivery System • Flexor Tendon • Growth Factors • Healing • Hyaluronic Acid • Lubricin • Rehabilitation

8.1
Introduction

A number of studies have shown that the risk of failure following intrasynovial flexor tendon transection is greatest in the early period after repair [1–4]. The factors that most often lead to a loss of function following tendon injury and repair are the development of repair site elongation and rupture and the formation of adhesions within the digital sheath. These complications are due primarily to the failure of the repair site to accrue strength within the first few weeks after suture repair, exacerbated by a post-traumatic increase in gliding resistance within the digital sheath [2, 4–6]. Research over the last 25 years has focused on mechanical and biological interventions to improve flexor tendon healing. Significant progress has been made in maintaining an effective gliding surface between the tendon and its sheath after surgical repair. However, less progress has

S. Thomopoulos (✉)
Orthopaedic Surgery and Biomedical Engineering, Washington University, St. Louis, MO, USA

A. Merolli, T.J. Joyce (eds), *Biomaterials in Hand Surgery.*
© Springer-Verlag Italia 2009

been made in improving the strength of the repair in the early post-operative period, leaving the tendon at risk for gap formation or even rupture.

An improved understanding of the reparative response of sutured intrasynovial flexor tendon has been achieved in recent years [7–11]. On tendon transection and repair, a clot forms between the tendon stumps and in the space between the gliding surface and the tendon sheath. Cellular elements within the clot release growth factors (e.g. platelet-derived growth factor (PDGF)-BB, interleukin growth factor) that induce and potentiate a localized inflammatory response. During the initial inflammatory phase, typically lasting less than 2 days, the wound is invaded by macrophages and other extrinsic cells, which secrete a second wave of growth factors capable of inducing neovascularization and initiating the reparative phase of repair. At 3 days, fibrinous tissue bridges the repair site. It is during this interval, at the earliest time points following repair, that adhesions have been noted to develop between the synovial lining of the tendon sheath and the gliding surface of the sutured tendon. From 4–7 days postinjury, during the proliferative and early reparative stages of healing, additional fibroblasts migrate into the wound, synthesizing type I collagen and forming an immature granulation tissue matrix. By 7 days, fibrin within the repair site serves as the initial scaffold of support for migrating epitenon cells [2]. The remodeling phase, 2–3 weeks post-repair, is marked by continued proliferation and migration of epitenon cells into the repair site and then by a gradual decrease in cellularity and an increase in collagen synthesis and cross-linking. By 17 days, the first blood vessels reach the repair site [12]. In the later stages, collagen is remodeled longitudinally and cross-linked within the extracellular matrix.

Manipulation of the mechanical environment post repair has led to significant improvements in the gliding properties (i.e. range of motion and tendon excursion) of the healing flexor tendon. These rehabilitation variables, however, have been unsuccessful in improving the strength of the repair, as the immature repair site has been unresponsive to either increasing levels of applied *in vivo* load or higher levels of intrasynovial repair site excursion [13–16]. Studies have suggested that future strategies for accelerating the repair process be directed toward altering the biological environment of the sutured tendon [7, 17–20]. A number of biomaterials have been proposed to enhance tendon gliding post repair, and to improve tendon strength through delivery of biofactors. Two general approaches have been taken for enhancing flexor tendon healing with biomaterials. In the first approach, tendons are coated with factors that improve the gliding properties of the tendon and/or suppress adhesion formation. Surface modifications include the use of natural (e.g. lubricin, hyaluronic acid) and synthetic (e.g. carbodiimide-derivatized hyaluronic acid) materials. In the second biological approach, growth factors, which are powerful regulators of biological function, are used to promote specific cellular activity. The patterns of natural expression of PDGF-BB, basic fibroblast growth factor (bFGF), transforming growth factor beta 1 (TGFβ1), and vascular endothelial growth factor (VEGF) vary dramatically over time during tendon healing [7]. Manipulation of the growth factor environment may lead to improved tendon healing. In the context of flexor tendon repair, increased matrix synthesis may lead to improved structural properties (e.g. strength), while increased hyaluroninc acid may lead to improved functional properties (e.g. range of

motion). In the following sections, prior results for mechanical and biological interventions to enhance flexor tendon healing will be reviewed.

8.2
Animal Models for Studying Flexor Tendon Injury and Repair

A number of animal models have been used to study intrasynovial flexor tendon injury
and repair. The two most commonly used models are the rabbit [21–38] and the canine
[4, 6, 13–16, 39–73]. As demonstrated by Potenza in 1962, the most clinically appropriate animal model for intrasynovial flexor tendon repair is the canine flexor tendon
model [69, 70]. Analysis of the flexor tendons and their surrounding structures demonstrated that the anatomy of the canine flexor tendon closely matches that of humans.
The flexor tendons in the dog are similar in size to the flexor tendons in humans, allowing the surgeon to use suture techniques similar to those used clinically. This animal
model has been used by a number of groups to evaluate rehabilitation variables, tendon
coatings, and growth factor treatments for tendon repair.

8.3
Mechanical Approaches for Enhanced Flexor Tendon Healing

It is well established that the mechanical loading environment (as determined by rehabilitation) post flexor tendon repair influences the healing process. The role of rehabilitation variables in modulating flexor tendon healing was recently reviewed by Boyer et
al [74]. While it has been known for many years that controlling the post-operative loading regimen is critical for preventing adhesions and promoting healing (Fig. 8.1) [39],
it is only recently that the variables of load magnitude and tendon excursion have been
critically and separately evaluated. Adhesion-free healing was demonstrated by a number of groups both experimentally and clinically, with passive and active motion rehabilitation [74]. However, results were mostly empirical and it was unclear whether the
reduction in adhesions was due to higher loads on the repair, or higher tendon excursion during the rehabilitation.

It is clear from *in vitro* and *in vivo* studies that tendon fibroblasts are responsive to
mechanical load. Both static and cyclic load have been shown to stimulate fibroblast
migration, fibroblast proliferation, and extracellular matrix synthesis. Hannafin et al
showed that load is necessary for tendon explants to maintain mechanical properties
[66]. Slack et al applied load to cultured flexor tendons and demonstrated increased
DNA and protein synthesis in loaded tendons [75]. The concept that mechanical load
can promote cellular activity and potentially improve flexor tendon healing was applied
by a number of groups in experimental and clinical studies. Small et al reported
improvements in clinical outcomes with active motion rehabilitation [76]. However,
this study also showed a 9% rupture rate, demonstrating the risks involved with high-load

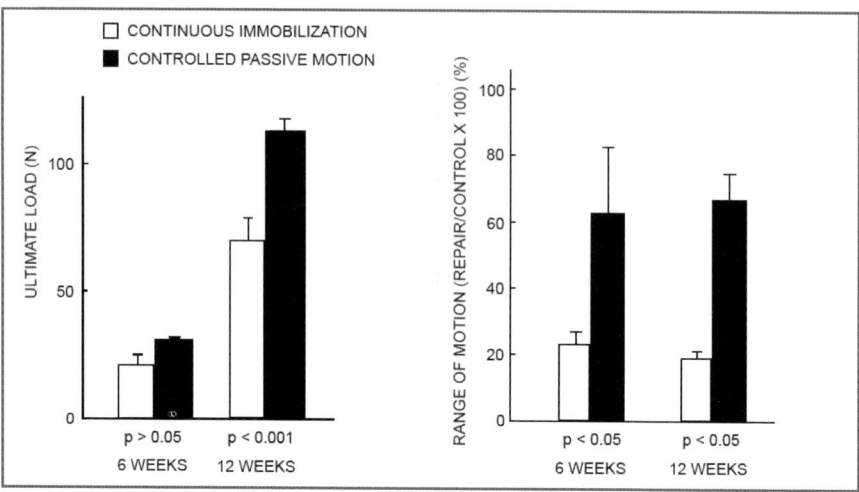

Fig. 8.1 Tensile properties (*left*) and gliding properties (*right*) were significantly better in the passive mobilization group compared to the immobilized group [39]. Error bars are standard error. Adapted from [39] with permission from Taylor and Francis Group

rehabilitation. The high rupture rate was likely due to the difficulty in controlling the load across the repair site during active motion. *In vivo* forces in one clinical study ranged from 1 N to 34 N for a passive digit flexion followed by an active tip pinch [77]. Therefore, while load does promote cell proliferation and matrix synthesis in a controlled environment, application of the concept to flexor tendon healing has proved difficult due to the increased risk of repair site gapping or rupture.

Passive motion rehabilitation (i.e. cyclic excursion of the tendon through the sheath at low loads) has also led to improvements in flexor tendon healing, primarily by preventing adhesion formation. In order to critically evaluate the role of loading versus tendon excursion, a series of studies was performed in the clinically appropriate canine model. The loads and excursion distances were first quantified for two rehabilitation protocols [14, 15, 39, 40, 78]. For low-load rehabilitation, the wrist was held in flexion and the digit was taken through flexion–extension passively. This resulted in less than 5 N of force across the repair site and 1.7 mm of tendon excursion. For high load rehabilitation, the wrist was held in extension and the digit was taken through flexion–extension passively. This resulted in 17 N of force across the repair site and 3.5 mm of tendon excursion. The authors found that the tensile properties did not differ between low- and high-force rehabilitation. Therefore, it is preferable to rehabilitate using a low-load regime and minimize the risk for gapping or rupture. There was also no difference between the low-excursion and the high-excursion groups when examining mechanical properties; both resulted in significantly fewer adhesions and improved gliding properties compared to immobilized tendons.

Based on the extensive literature examining rehabilitation variables for flexor tendon repair, a passive motion protocol should be used that emphasizes tendon excursion through the sheath rather than high force across the repair. Manipulation of the mechanical environment post-operatively has successfully reduced ruptures and has minimized adhesions formation in the early period after repair. However, even with established rehabilitation techniques, the tendon is still at significant risk for rupture and adhesions in the first 3 weeks after repair. As mechanical approaches for improving the repair have been exhausted, future strategies must incorporate biological and bio-material interventions for enhancing flexor tendon repair. As outlined in the next sections, these research approaches are currently focused on two areas: (1) coating or treating the surface of the tendon to improve gliding properties; and (2) delivering growth factors to the repair site in an effort to enhance matrix synthesis and improve both gliding and tensile properties.

8.4
Biomaterials for Enhanced Flexor Tendon Gliding

Gliding of the tendon within its sheath is critical for digital function. The low-friction contact that exists in uninjured tissue is primarily determined by the lubricants hyaluronic acid and lubricin. One study demonstrated that the gliding resistance at the interface between the tendon and its sheath increased significantly after the tendon had been treated with a hyaluronidase solution (i.e. after the hyaluronic acid was stripped from the tissue surfaces) [79]. The authors proposed that hyaluronidase-sensitive materials, such as hyaluronic acid, may act as boundary lubricants, facilitating gliding and reducing the resistance between the tendon and its sheath. A separate study showed that phospholipids, hyaluronic acid, and protein components are all involved in maintaining the low gliding resistance of flexor tendons [62]. More recently, lubricin has been identified on the surface of flexor tendons [59, 60]. Lubricin was found both on the tendon surface and at the interface of collagen fiber bundles within the tendon. Lubricin has many distinct biological functions, including lubrication, anti-adhesion, and regulation of cell growth. It may therefore play an important role in tendon gliding and in adhesion formation after tendon repair.

   Surgical repair of intrasynovial flexor tendons can result in fibrous adhesions, gaps between the repaired tendon ends, and suture knots, all of which will increase the friction between the tendon and its sheath. In order to reduce this friction and improve the gliding properties of the tendon (and hence improve digital function), a number of bio-materials have been utilized [36–38, 54, 55, 59–64, 79, 80–86]. The most studied lubricating biomaterial for flexor tendon repair is hyaluronic acid. Initial *in vivo* studies using hyaluronic acid to enhance the gliding properties of the repaired tendon were difficult to interpret [22, 26, 84, 87–89]. However, most studies showed some benefit for tendon gliding due to hyaluronic acid. One *in vitro* study demonstrated that explanted tendons treated with hyaluronic acid had better gliding properties than untreated tendons [54]. The excursion resistance between the tendon and its sheath was evaluated in tendons which were soaked in hyaluronic acid for five minutes, and compared to contralateral untreated tendons. The authors demonstrated that the gliding resistance of tendons was significantly decreased after the administration of hyaluronic acid, suggesting that the administration of hyaluronic acid may improve the gliding function of a flexor tendon graft *in vivo*. These results were also reproduced in flexor tendon *in vitro* repairs [57]. The concept of improved gliding using hyaluronic acid was tested in an *in vivo* canine model by a different research group [84]. The authors demonstrated with gross and histological evidence that hyaluronic acid had a beneficial effect on both the repair site and the synovial sheath by decreasing the peripheral inflammatory response and promoting contact healing between the repaired tendon ends.

More recently, it has been proposed that proper attachment of hyaluronic acid to tendon is critical for providing a long-lasting gliding surface between two tissues. The inconsistent results in prior literature of studies attempting to use hyaluronic acid to improve flexor tendon healing were likely due to rapid clearing of the material from the wound site. In a number of studies, carbodiimide derivatization was used to modify hyaluronic acid (cd-HA), allowing the authors to chemically bind hyaluronic acid to exposed amino groups, such as those in the collagenous tendon matrix (Fig. 8.2) [55, 61, 80–83, 85]. cd-HA is less soluble in water than normal hyaluronic acid and is thought to increase the binding strength of the hyaluronic acid to collagen. The derivatized biomaterial therefore has longer residence time than the unmodified biomaterial, and may be more effective in improving the gliding properties of healing flexor tendons [61, 90]. Yang et al examined the effect of cd-HA gel on gliding during cyclic loading of a repaired tendon *in vitro* [85]. Flexor digitorum profundus tendons were divided into three groups: control, unmodified hyaluronic acid, and cd-HA. The gliding resistance was measured before laceration and after suture repair. From the 50th

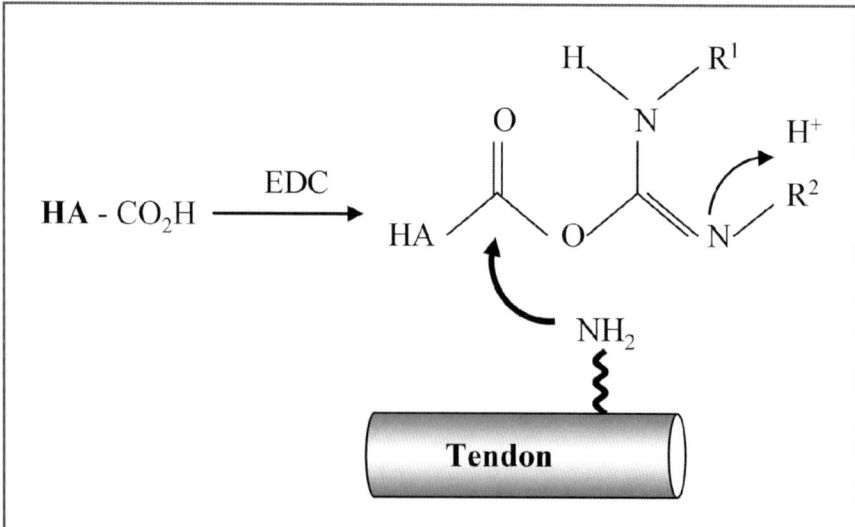

Fig. 8.2 Carboxyl groups in the hyaluronic acid (HA) are activated by 1-ethyl-3-(3-dimethylaminopropyl) carbodiimide hydrochloride (EDC) to form O-acylisoureas, which bind to the amino groups on the tendon surface. Adapted from [61], with permission from The Journal of Bone and Joint Surgery, Inc.

loading cycle onwards, gliding resistance was significantly lower in the cd-HA gel group than in the control group. Zhao et al tested this biomaterial *in vivo* for flexor tendon healing [61]. They hypothesized that surface modification of an extrasynovial tendon with the use of cd-HA will improve gliding ability and digital function after tendon grafting in a canine model *in vivo*. The peroneus longus tendon was harvested and transplanted to replace the flexor digitorum profundus tendon. Peroneus longus tendons were coated with cd-HA or immersed in saline solution. Gliding resistance of the cd-HA group was significantly lower than that of the saline group (Fig. 8.3). The authors concluded that treating the surface of an extrasynovial tendon autograft with a cd-HA–gelatin polymer may improve tendon gliding and improve the quality of tendon graft surgery.

Moro-oka et al showed that phospholipids may also facilitate tendon gliding [31]. Dipalmitoyl phosphatidylcholine, a phospholipid that may provide boundary lubrication in synovial joints, was examined for flexor tendon repair. In a set of *in vitro* experiments, the authors showed that the frictional coefficient of tendons treated with a combination of dipalmitoyl phosphatidylcholine and hyaluronic acid was lower than if they were treated with saline solution or hyaluronic acid. In a set of *in vivo* experiments using a rabbit animal model, flexor digitorum fibularis tendons were injured, repaired, and treated with either saline solution, hyaluronic acid, or a mixture of dipalmitoyl phosphatidylcholine and hyaluronic acid. The work required to break adhesions post repair and healing was significantly greater for the tendons that had been treated with

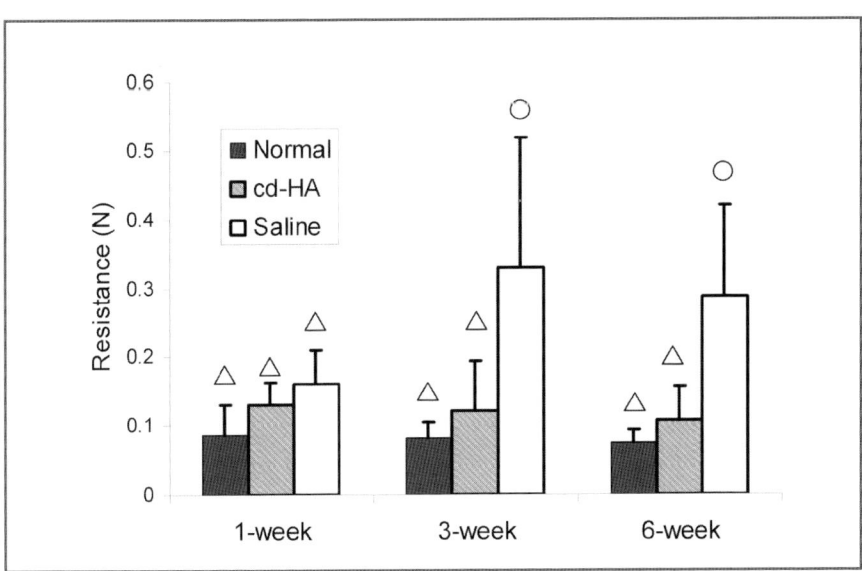

Fig. 8.3 The gliding resistance in the cd-HA-treated tendons was similar to normal and significantly lower than the saline-treated tendons 3 and 6 weeks after the repair [61]. A difference in symbols denotes a significant difference between values (p < 0.05), with the triangle being significantly less than the circle. Adapted from [61], with permission from The Journal of Bone and Joint Surgery, Inc.

saline solution compared to those treated with dipalmitoyl phosphatidylcholine and hyaluronic acid. The *in vitro* and *in vivo* results of this study demonstrate that the administration of a phospholipid/hyaluronic acid coating may improve tendon lubrication, prevent adhesion formation, and improve hand function after tendon repair.

Recent work has examined the effect of exogenous lubricin for improving tendon gliding. Following the approach taken with hyaluronic acid, Taguchi et al modified the surfaces of repaired flexor tendons with lubricin, and determined the effect on tendon gliding *in vitro* [63]. Canine flexor digitorum tendons were lacerated, repaired, and treated with various surface modifications, including attachment of lubricin. After treatment, gliding resistance was measured under simulated flexion/extension motion. Surface modification significantly improved gliding properties. Scanning electron microscopy showed that treated tendons had smoother surfaces after cyclic loading that untreated tendons, which appeared roughened. There was a trend suggesting than lubricin fixed on the tendon may provide additional improvements to gliding over that provided by cd-HA alone. Similar results were reported for extrasynovial tendons tested *in vitro* [64]. Future work must examine the effect of lubricin surface modification on the gliding properties of repaired flexor tendons *in vivo*.

8.5
Biomaterials for Growth Factor-enhanced Flexor Tendon Healing

Growth factors, synthesized naturally or administered therapeutically, are powerful regulators of biological function [56, 91–94]. The patterns of natural expression of PDGF-BB, bFGF, TGFβ1, and VEGF vary dramatically over time during tendon healing [7]. Endogenous release of these factors following injury and repair are not adequate to restore a healing tendon's structural properties to levels approaching pre-injury status. Manipulation of the growth factor environment, therefore, has been an important strategy for improving the strength and stiffness of repaired tendon and ligament, with PDGF-BB, bFGF and TGFβ1 showing promise for stimulating collagen synthesis and increasing the stiffness and strength of the repair site [93, 95, 96]. In recent studies on tendon [18] and ligament [97] repair, bFGF was effective in promoting cellular proliferation, neovascularization, collagen production, and collagen organization. In another study, high doses of exogenous PDGF-BB, delivered in a fibrin sealant, led to substantial increases in ultimate load and energy absorbed to failure following ligament repair *in vivo* [98]. However, these studies and others indicate that dosage, time of administration, residence time, and synergistic effects significantly complicate the use of growth factors, and improved mechanical properties have not always been seen following their administration. In addition, studies utilizing some factors (e.g. TGFβ1) indicate that adhesion formation around the repair site may be stimulated following growth factor delivery [27].

Administration of growth factors by bolus injection has been shown to result in significant fluctuations in local tissue and serum concentrations, with removal from the repair site, denaturation, and clearance from the circulation occurring within 48 hours

[99]. Recent studies have shown that binding a cytokine to a biocompatible matrix can prolong its elimination half-life, extending its effects. Degradable polyethylene glycol hydromatrices, polylactic-co-glycololic acid and gelatin microspheres, rapidly resorbing calcium phosphate pastes, collagen, and alginate matrices have been used effectively to suppress the initial burst of growth factor administration, providing sustained release for as long as 8 weeks following administration [100, 101]. *In vitro* and *in vivo* studies have shown that sustained delivery can be highly effective when compared to bolus administration and to controls. Sustained delivery at the repaired flexor tendon may be especially beneficial, as the fibroblasts that mount the healing response do not infiltrate the wound site until 2–3 days after injury. Growth factors delivered with a bolus injection at the time of injury would be cleared before they could stimulate the cells of interest.

A number of biomaterials have been used to deliver growth factors to musculoskeletal tissues. Burdick et al, using degradable polyethylene glycol hydromatrices as delivery vehicles for administering osteoinductive growth factors, demonstrated the ability to control protein release, and achieve improved gene expression for osteocalcin and collagen, and increased mineralization compared to control [102]. Lam et al, using polylactic co-glycolic acid microspheres, limited initial growth factor bolus administration to less than 1%, controlled nerve growth factor release effectively over time, and demonstrated improved nerve regeneration *in vivo* [103]. Azuma et al prevented tendon graft deterioration post-transplantation with the delayed administration of TGFβ1 and epidermal growth factor (EGF) compared to the early administration of these growth factors [104], and Tabata et al, using bFGF-impregnated biodegradable gelatin microspheres, showed significantly enhanced vascularization *in vivo*, compared to control [105]. A number of other investigators have demonstrated similar effects in other tissues with the use of systems designed to control growth factor administration over time [11, 98, 101, 106–113].

A novel growth factor delivery system was developed recently by Sakiyama-Elbert and colleagues, which provides for sustained administration by immobilizing high-affinity heparin-binding growth factors, protecting them from degradation during the early intervals following delivery [114]. The delivery system, designed to mimic the extracellular matrix, allows release of growth factors from a three-dimensional fibrin matrix in an active, cell-mediated manner – one that responds to the naturally occurring cellular activity associated with repair (Fig. 8.4) [51, 115]. A bi-domain peptide was used with a Factor XIIIa substrate from α2 plasmin inhibitor at the N-terminus of the peptide to allow covalent cross-linking to fibrin during polymerization. The peptide C-terminus contained a heparin-binding domain similar to that from anti-thrombin III. This domain allowed the non-covalent immobilization of heparin to the fibrin matrix. The heparin can in turn bind heparin-binding growth factors, such as PDGF-BB, and prevent them from diffusing out of the fibrin matrix. Release of growth factor from the matrix occurs via three mechanisms: (1) dissociation of growth factor from matrix-bound heparin and subsequent diffusion of free heparin-binding growth factor; (2) proteolytic degradation of the fibrin matrix; or (3) enzymatic degradation of heparin.

Using this delivery system, recent *in vitro* reports showed that the release kinetics of PDGF-BB could be modulated by varying the ratio of PDGF-BB to heparin (Fig. 8.5) [51, 116]. In the presence of canine tendon fibroblasts, the delivery system

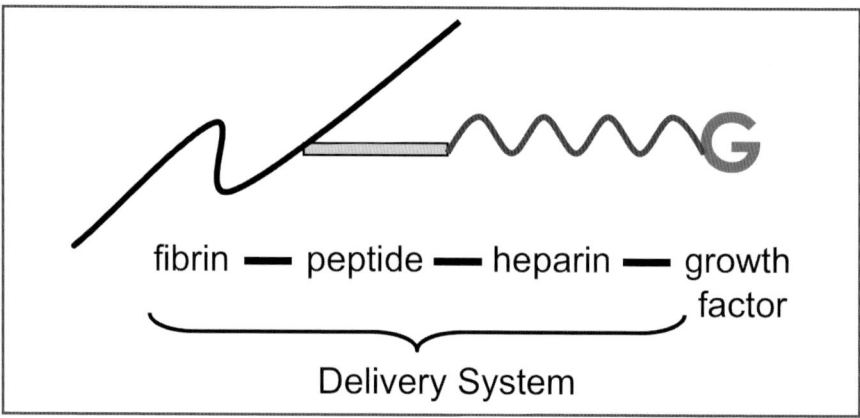

Fig. 8.4 A fibrin-based delivery system was designed to administer PDGF-BB in a manner that was tailored specifically to the temporal progression of tissue regeneration [51]. The N-terminus of the peptide was covalently cross-linked to fibrin during polymerization. The C-terminus of the peptide contained a heparin-binding domain. This domain allowed the non-covalent immobilization of heparin to the fibrin matrix. The heparin in turn trapped the heparin-binding growth factor PDGF-BB, preventing it from diffusing out of the fibrin matrix. Adapted from [51] ©2007, with permission of John Wiley & Sons, Inc.

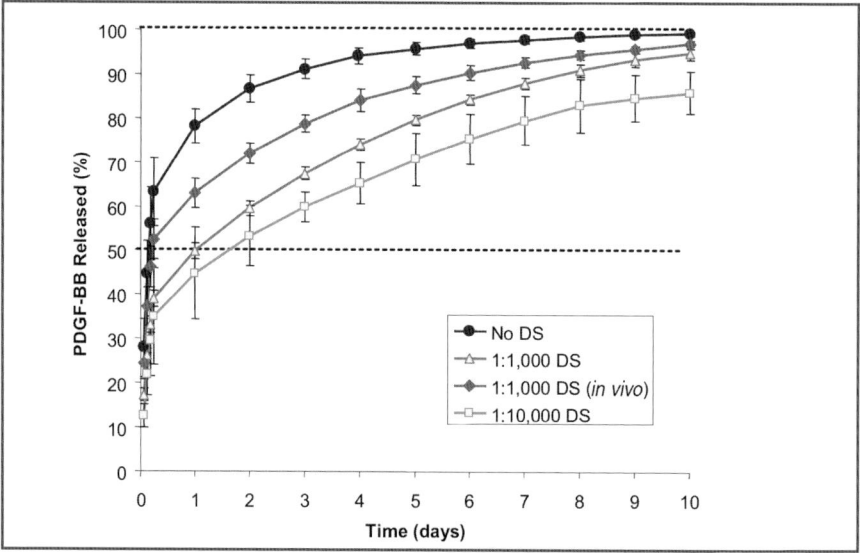

Fig. 8.5 Sustained release was achieved through the use of a fibrin matrix delivery system (DS) [51]. The slowest release was achieved using a 1:10,000 growth factor to heparin ratio. All groups were significantly different from each other at times 3 through 6 days. The 1:1,000 and the 1:10,000 groups were significantly different from the other two groups at times 1 through 9 days. Note that the "1:1,000 DS (*in vivo*)" group represents a delivery system formulation identical to that used for the *in vivo* studies. Error bars are standard deviation. Adapted from [51] ©2007, with permission of John Wiley & Sons, Inc.

prolonged the duration of PDGF-BB release from fibrin matrices, thus demonstrating that cells are able to liberate PDGF-BB retained by the delivery system. Sustained delivery of PDGF-BB promoted increased cell proliferation and collagen synthesis compared to fibrin without delivery system. The responding cells in the *in vitro* system were canine fibroblasts isolated from the same region as those used in previous *in vivo* flexor tendon repair studies. Therefore, through the use of growth factors, it may be possible to modulate the rate of cell proliferation and extracellular matrix synthesis *in vivo*, to enhance and accelerate the tendon healing process.

The *in vitro* results were confirmed *in vivo* using the canine intrasynovial flexor tendon model [51]. Delivery of PDGF-BB *in vivo* led to a qualitative increase in cell density, cell proliferation, and type I collagen mRNA expression. PDGF-BB also led to statistically significant increases in total DNA and reducible collagen crosslinks. As the tendon is most vulnerable to rupture in the first weeks after surgical repair, acceleration of the repair process without adhesion formation is a primary goal in treating flexor tendon injuries. The most dramatic changes in cell proliferation and matrix synthesis in this study occurred at the earliest time point studied, implying that healing was accelerated early in the repair process by PDGF-BB delivery.

A subsequent study examined whether the increased biological activity due to PDGF-BB would lead to improvements in the function and strength of the tendon repair [49]. At three weeks of healing, proximal interphalangeal joint and distal interphalangeal joint rotation values were significantly higher for the PDGF-BB-treated tendons compared to the repair-alone tendons (Fig. 8.6). Excursion values were also significantly higher in the PDGF-BB treated tendons (Fig. 8.6). This study demonstrated that the gliding properties of repaired flexor tendons were significantly improved due

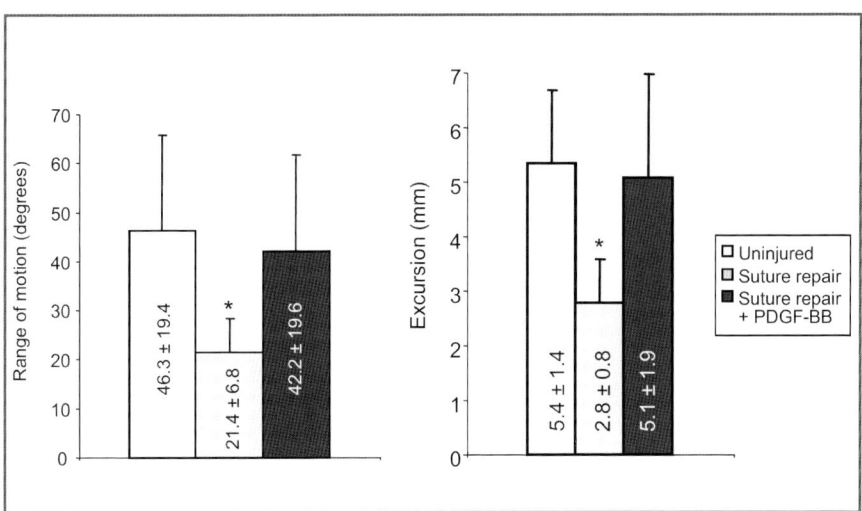

Fig. 8.6 Range of motion and tendon excursion were significantly improved due to PDGF-BB treatment (*p < 0.05) [49]. Error bars are standard deviation. Adapted from [49], with permission from Elsevier

to the sustained administration of PDGF-BB. Other studies have shown that PDGF-BB stimulates hyaluronic acid biosynthesis in animal fibroblasts *in vivo* and human fibroblasts *in vitro* [117–125]. As described in earlier sections, hyaluronic acid is normally found on the surface of intrasynovial tendons and serves as a lubricant. The addition of hyaluronic acid to flexor tendon repair improves the gliding properties of the tendon during healing. In one study, PDGF-BB stimulated normal human mesothelial cells to synthesize hyaluronic acid which, when extruded from cells, formed hyaluronan-containing pellicular matrices or coats [119]. In the *in vivo* flexor tendon repair study, the sustained delivery of PDGF-BB led to improved tendon gliding, possibly through a stimulation of hyaluronic acid synthesis. However, this study did not demonstrate any significant differences in tensile properties when comparing PDGF-BB to repair-alone tendons. The failure to achieve improvements in ultimate load, stiffness, and strain in the experimental group may have been due to suboptimal PDGF-BB dosage, or suboptimal release kinetics. Improvements in mechanical properties may also be seen with the delivery of additional factors in combination with PDGF-BB. While PDGF-BB is a promising growth factor for tendon repair based on its ability to stimulate fibroblast proliferation and matrix synthesis, the addition of growth factors such as bFGF or TGFβ1, alone or in combination with PDGF-BB, may produce better results.

A different approach was taken by Hamada et al to deliver bFGF for flexor tendon repair [126]. The authors developed a nylon suture that was able to release various growth factors directly to the repair. Sutures were coated with cross-linked gelatin and soaked in bFGF. Sustained release of the growth factor using this biomaterial was achieved for up to 3 weeks. A rabbit model was used to assess the effect of these coated sutures for tendon repair. There was an apparent fibroblastic response to the coated sutures, and the ultimate load in the treated group was significantly increased at 3 weeks after surgery. The authors concluded that a bFGF-coated nylon suture can be used to enhance flexor tendon healing.

Summary

⟩ Based on extensive work in the canine model and in clinical studies, it is clear that passive (i.e., low-load) motion should be utilized after primary intrasynovial flexor tendon repair. This rehabilitation approach minimizes adhesion formation and protects the repair from rupture. However, even with these advances in rehabilitation, flexor tendon repairs are still at risk for adhesions, gapping, and rupture in the early period after surgical repair. Current trends in flexor tendon research demonstrate great promise for further improving the outcome after surgical repair. Biomaterial coatings for flexor tendons can improve tendon gliding and digital function more than rehabilitation alone. Growth factors, delivered in a sustained manner using novel biomaterials, can stimulate tendon fibroblasts to proliferate and produce the appropriate extracellular matrix, improving the strength of the repair. Future studies will translate these basic science studies from animal models to the clinic, for enhanced flexor tendon healing.

References

1. Beredjiklian PK (2003) Biologic aspects of flexor tendon laceration and repair. J Bone Joint Surg Am. American Volume 85-A:539–550.
2. Gelberman RH, Vandeberg JS, Manske PR, Akeson WH (1985) The early stages of flexor tendon healing: a morphologic study of the first fourteen days. J Hand Surg Am 10:776–784.
3. Tanaka T, Amadio PC, Zhao C, Zobitz ME, Yang C, An KN (2004) Gliding characteristics and gap formation for locking and grasping tendon repairs: a biomechanical study in a human cadaver model. J Hand Surg 29:6–14.
4. Zhao C, Amadio PC, Paillard P et al (2004) Digital resistance and tendon strength during the first week after flexor digitorum profundus tendon repair in a canine model in vivo. J Bone Joint Surg Am 86-A:320–327.
5. Khan U, Kakar S, Akali A et al (2000) Modulation of the formation of adhesions during the healing of injured tendons. J Bone Joint Surg Am 82:1054–1058.
6. Gelberman RH, Boyer MI, Brodt MD et al (1999) The effect of gap formation at the repair site on the strength and excursion of intrasynovial flexor tendons. An experimental study on the early stages of tendon-healing in dogs. J Bone Joint Surg Am 81:975–982.
7. Molloy T, Wang Y, Murrell G (2003) The roles of growth factors in tendon and ligament healing. Sports Medicine 33:381–394.
8. Albright J (1987) The scientific basis of orthopaedics. Appleton and Lange, Norwalk, CT.
9. Mast BA (1997) Healing in other tissues. Surgical Clinics of North America 77:529–547.
10. Hyman J, Rodeo SA (2000) Injury and repair of tendons and ligaments. Physical Medicine and Rehabilitation Clinics of North America 11:267–288.
11. Woo SL, Hildebrand K, Watanabe N et al (1999) Tissue engineering of ligament and tendon healing. Clin Orthop Relat Res 367(suppl):S312–323.
12. Gelberman RH, Khabie V, Cahill CJ (1991) The revascularization of healing flexor tendons in the digital sheath. A vascular injection study in dogs. J Bone Joint Surg Am 73:868–881
13. Silva MJ, Brodt MD, Boyer MI et al (1999) Effects of increased in vivo excursion on digital range of motion and tendon strength following flexor tendon repair. J Orthop Res 17:777–783.
14. Lieber RL, Amiel D, Kaufman KR et al (1996) Relationship between joint motion and flexor tendon force in the canine forelimb. J Hand Surg Am 21:957–962.
15. Lieber RL, Silva MJ, Amiel D, Gelberman RH (1999) Wrist and digital joint motion produce unique flexor tendon force and excursion in the canine forelimb. J Biomech 32:175–181.
16. Boyer MI, Gelberman RH, Burns ME et al (2001) Intrasynovial flexor tendon repair. An experimental study comparing low and high levels of in vivo force during rehabilitation in canines. J Bone Joint Surg Am 83-A:891–899.
17. Chan BP, Chan KM, Maffulli N et al (1997) Effect of basic fibroblast growth factor. An in vitro study of tendon healing. Clin Orthop Relat Res 342:239–247.
18. Chan BP, Fu S, Qin L et al (2000) Effects of basic fibroblast growth factor (bFGF) on early stages of tendon healing: a rat patellar tendon model. Acta Orthopaedica Scandinavica 71:513–518.
19. Chang J, Thunder R, Most D et al (2000) Studies in flexor tendon wound healing: neutralizing antibody to TGF-beta1 increases postoperative range of motion. Plastic and Reconstructive Surgery 105:148–155.
20. Yoshikawa Y, Abrahamsson SO (2001) Dose-related cellular effects of platelet-derived growth factor-BB differ in various types of rabbit tendons in vitro. Acta Orthopaedica Scandinavica 72:287–292.
21. Matthews P, Richards H (1974) The repair potential of digital flexor tendons. An experimental study. Journal of Bone and Joint Surgery. British Volume 56-B:618–625.

22. Thomas SC, Jones LC, Hungerford DS (1986) Hyaluronic acid and its effect on postoperative adhesions in the rabbit flexor tendon. A preliminary look. Clin Orthop Relat Res 206:281–289.

23. Daniel JC, Mills DK (1988) Proteoglycan synthesis by cells cultured from regions of the rabbit flexor tendon. Connective Tissue Research 17:215–230.

24. Abrahamsson SO, Lundborg G, Lohmander LS (1989) Tendon healing in vivo. An experimental model. Scandinavian Journal of Plastic and Reconstructive Surgery and Hand Surgery 23:199–205.

25. Abrahamsson SO, Lundborg G, Lohmander LS (1991) Long-term explant culture of rabbit flexor tendon: effects of recombinant human insulin-like growth factor-I and serum on matrix metabolism. J Orthop Res 9:503–515.

26. Salti NI, Tuel RJ, Mass DP (1993) Effect of hyaluronic acid on rabbit profundus flexor tendon healing in vitro. Journal of Surgical Research 55:411–415.

27. Chang J, Most D, Stelnicki E et al (1997) Gene expression of transforming growth factor beta-1 in rabbit zone II flexor tendon wound healing: evidence for dual mechanisms of repair. Plastic and Reconstructive Surgery 100:937–944.

28. Chang J, Most D, Thunder R et al (1998) Molecular studies in flexor tendon wound healing: the role of basic fibroblast growth factor gene expression. J Bone Joint Surg Am 23:1052–1058.

29. Moro-oka T, Miura H, Higaki H et al (1999) A new friction tester of the flexor tendon. J Biomech 32:1131–1134.

30. Chang J, Thunder R, Most D et al (2000) Studies in flexor tendon wound healing: neutralizing antibody to TGF-beta1 increases postoperative range of motion. Plastic and Reconstructive Surgery 105:148–155.

31. Moro-oka T, Miura H, Mawatari T et al (2000) Mixture of hyaluronic acid and phospholipid prevents adhesion formation on the injured flexor tendon in rabbits. J Orthop Res 18:835–840.

32. Ngo M, Pham H, Longaker MT, Chang J (2001) Differential expression of transforming growth factor-beta receptors in a rabbit zone II flexor tendon wound healing model. Plastic and Reconstructive Surgery 108:1260–1267.

33. Klein MB, Yalamanchi N, Pham H et al (2002) Flexor tendon healing in vitro: effects of TGF-beta on tendon cell collagen production. J Bone Joint Surg Am 27:615–620.

34. Zhang AY, Pham H, Ho F et al (2004) Inhibition of TGF-beta-induced collagen production in rabbit flexor tendons. J Hand Surg Am 29:230–235.

35. Mehta V, Kang Q, Luo J et al (2005) Characterization of adenovirus-mediated gene transfer in rabbit flexor tendons. J Hand Surg Am 30:136–141.

36. Namba J, Shimada K, Saito M et al (2007) Modulation of peritendinous adhesion formation by alginate solution in a rabbit flexor tendon model. J Biomed Mater Res B Appl Biomater 80:273–279.

37. de Wit T, de Putter D, Tra WM et al (2008) Auto-crosslinked hyaluronic acid gel accelerates healing of rabbit flexor tendons in vivo. J Orthop Res 28 August, epub ahead of print.

38. Liu Y, Skardal A, Shu XZ, Prestwich GD (2008) Prevention of peritendinous adhesions using a hyaluronan-derived hydrogel film following partial-thickness flexor tendon injury. J Orthop Res 26:562–569.

39. Woo SL, Gelberman RH, Cobb NG et al (1981) The importance of controlled passive mobilization on flexor tendon healing. A biomechanical study. Acta Orthopaedica Scandinavica 52:615–622.

40. Gelberman RH, Woo SL, Lothringer K et al (1982) Effects of early intermittent passive mobilization on healing canine flexor tendons. J Bone Joint Surg Am 7:170–175.

41. Duffy FJ, Jr., Seiler JG, Gelberman RH, Hergrueter CA (1995) Growth factors and canine flexor tendon healing: initial studies in uninjured and repair models. J Bone Joint Surg Am 20:645–649.

42. Ridder M, Towler DA, Gelberman RH, Boyer MI (2000) Expression of mRNA for vascular endothelial growth factor at the repair site of healing canine flexor tendon. J Orthop Res 18:247–252.

43. Silva MJ, Boyer MI, Ditsios K et al (2002) The insertion site of the canine flexor digitorum profundus tendon heals slowly following injury and suture repair. J Orthop Res 20:447–453.

44. Ditsios K, Leversedge FJ, Gelberman RH et al (2003) Neovascularization of the flexor digitorum profundus tendon after avulsion injury: an in vivo canine study. J Bone Joint Surg Am 28:231–236.

45. Boyer MI, Harwood F, Ditsios K et al (2003) Two-portal repair of canine flexor tendon insertion site injuries: histologic and immunohistochemical characterization of healing during the early postoperative period. J Bone Joint Surg Am 28:469–474.

46. Ditsios K, Boyer MI, Kusano N et al (2003) Bone loss following tendon laceration, repair and passive mobilization. J Orthop Res 21:990–996.

47. Thomopoulos S, Harwood FL, Silva MJ et al (2005) Effect of several growth factors on canine flexor tendon fibroblast proliferation and collagen synthesis in vitro. J Hand Surg Am 30:441–447.

48. Silva MJ, Thomopoulos S, Kusano N et al (2006) Early healing of flexor tendon insertion site injuries: Tunnel repair is mechanically and histologically inferior to surface repair in a canine model. J Orthop Res 24:990–1000.

49. Gelberman RH, Thomopoulos S, Sakiyama-Elbert SE et al (2007) The early effects of sustained platelet-derived growth factor administration on the functional and structural properties of repaired intrasynovial flexor tendons: an in vivo biomechanic study at 3 weeks in canines. J Hand Surg Am 32:373–379.

50. Thomopoulos S, Matsuzaki H, Zaegel M et al (2007) Alendronate prevents bone loss and improves tendon-to-bone repair strength in a canine model. J Orthop Res 25:473–479.

51. Thomopoulos S, Zaegel M, Das R et al (2007) PDGF-BB released in tendon repair using a novel delivery system promotes cell proliferation and collagen remodeling. J Orthop Res 25:1358–1368.

52. Thomopoulos S, Zampiakis E, Das R et al (2008) The effect of muscle loading on flexor tendon-to-bone healing in a canine model. J Orthop Res 26:1611–1617.

53. Okuda Y, Gorski JP, An KN, Amadio PC (1987) Biochemical, histological, and biomechanical analyses of canine tendon. J Orthop Res 5:60–68.

54. Nishida J, Araki S, Akasaka T et al (2004) Effect of hyaluronic acid on the excursion resistance of tendon grafts. A biomechanical study in a canine model in vitro. Journal of Bone and Joint Surgery. British Volume 86:918–924.

55. Sun YL, Yang C, Amadio PC et al (2004) Reducing friction by chemically modifying the surface of extrasynovial tendon grafts. J Orthop Res 22:984–989.

56. Tsubone T, Moran SL, Amadio PC et al (2004) Expression of growth factors in canine flexor tendon after laceration in vivo. Annals of Plastic Surgery 53:393–397.

57. Akasaka T, Nishida J, Araki S et al (2005) Hyaluronic acid diminishes the resistance to excursion after flexor tendon repair: an in vitro biomechanical study. J Biomech 38:503–507.

58. Tanaka T, Amadio PC, Zhao C et al (2005) Effect of elbow position on canine flexor digitorum profundus tendon tension. J Orthop Res 23:249–253.

59. Sun Y, Berger EJ, Zhao C et al (2006) Mapping lubricin in canine musculoskeletal tissues. Connective Tissue Research 47:215–221.

60. Sun Y, Berger EJ, Zhao C et al (2006) Expression and mapping of lubricin in canine flexor tendon. J Orthop Res 24:1861–1868.

61. Zhao C, Sun YL, Amadio PC et al (2006) Surface treatment of flexor tendon autografts with carbodiimide-derivatized hyaluronic Acid. An in vivo canine model. J Bone Joint Surg Am 88:2181–2191.

62. Sun Y, Chen MY, Zhao C et al (2008) The effect of hyaluronidase, phospholipase, lipid solvent and trypsin on the lubrication of canine flexor digitorum profundus tendon. J Orthop Res 26:1225–1229.

63. Taguchi M, Sun YL, Zhao C et al (2008) Lubricin surface modification improves tendon gliding after tendon repair in a canine model in vitro. J Orthop Res 6 August 2008, epub ahead of print.

64. Taguchi M, Sun YL, Zhao C et al (2008) Lubricin surface modification improves extrasynovial tendon gliding in a canine model in vitro. J Bone Joint Surg Am 90:129–135.

65. Potenza AD, Herte MC (1982) The synovial cavity as a "tissue culture in situ" – science or nonsense? J Bone Joint Surg Am 7:196–199.

66. Hannafin JA, Arnoczky SP, Hoonjan A, Torzilli PA (1995) Effect of stress deprivation and cyclic tensile loading on the material and morphologic properties of canine flexor digitorum profundus tendon: an in vitro study. J Orthop Res 13:907–914.

67. Ritty TM, Herzog J (2003) Tendon cells produce gelatinases in response to type I collagen attachment. J Orthop Res 21:442–450.

68. Baker AR, Abreu EL, Mascha E, Derwin KA (2004) Homotypic variation of canine flexor tendons: implications for the design of experimental studies in animal models. J Biomech 37:959–968.

69. Potenza AD (1962) Detailed evaluation of healing processes in canine flexor digital tendons. Military Medicine 127:34–47.

70. Potenza AD (1962) Tendon healing within the flexor digital sheath in the dog. J Bone Joint Surg Am 44-A:49–64.

71. Potenza AD (1963) Critical evaluation of flexor-tendon healing and adhesion formation within artificial digital sheaths. J Bone Joint Surg Am 45:1217–1233.

72. Potenza AD (1964) The Healing of Autogenous Tendon Grafts within the Flexor Digital Sheath in Dogs. J Bone Joint Surg Am 46:1462–1484.

73. Potenza AD (1964) Prevention of Adhesions to Healing Digital Flexor Tendons. JAMA 187:187–191.

74. Boyer MI, Goldfarb CA, Gelberman RH (2005) Recent progress in flexor tendon healing. The modulation of tendon healing with rehabilitation variables. Journal of Hand Therapy 18:80–85; quiz 86.

75. Slack C, Flint MH, Thompson BM (1984) The effect of tensional load on isolated embryonic chick tendons in organ culture. Connective Tissue Research 12:229–247.

76. Small JO, Brennen MD, Colville J (1989) Early active mobilisation following flexor tendon repair in zone 2. J Hand Surg Am (Edinburgh, Scotland) 14:383–391.

77. Schuind F, Garcia-Elias M, Cooney WP, 3rd, An KN (1992) Flexor tendon forces: in vivo measurements. J Hand Surg Am 17:291–298.

78. Takai S, Woo SL, Horibe S, Tung DK, Gelberman RH (1991) The effects of frequency and duration of controlled passive mobilization on tendon healing. J Orthop Res 9:705–713.

79. Uchiyama S, Amadio PC, Ishikawa J, An KN (1997) Boundary lubrication between the tendon and the pulley in the finger. J Bone Joint Surg Am 79:213–218.

80. Momose T, Amadio PC, Sun YL et al (2002) Surface modification of extrasynovial tendon by chemically modified hyaluronic acid coating. J Biomed Mater Res 59:219–224.

81. Tanaka T, Sun YL, Zhao C et al (2006) Optimization of surface modifications of extrasynovial tendon to improve its gliding ability in a canine model in vitro. J Orthop Res 24:1555–1561.

82. Tanaka T, Sun YL, Zhao C et al (2006) Effect of curing time and concentration for a chemical treatment that improves surface gliding for extrasynovial tendon grafts in vitro. J Biomed Mater Res. Part A 79:451–455.

83. Tanaka T, Zhao C, Sun YL et al (2007) The effect of carbodiimide-derivatized hyaluronic acid and gelatin surface modification on peroneus longus tendon graft in a short-term canine model in vivo. J Hand Surg Am 32:876–881.

84. Amiel D, Ishizue K, Billings E, Jr. et al (1989) Hyaluronan in flexor tendon repair. J Hand Surg Am 14:837–843.

85. Yang C, Amadio PC, Sun YL et al (2004) Tendon surface modification by chemically modified HA coating after flexor digitorum profundus tendon repair. J Biomed Mater Res B Appl Biomater 68:15–20.

86. McCombe D, Kubicki M, Witschi C et al (2006) A collagen prolyl 4-hydroxylase inhibitor reduces adhesions after tendon injury. Clin Orthop Relat Res 451:251–256.

87. Hagberg L (1992) Exogenous hyaluronate as an adjunct in the prevention of adhesions after flexor tendon surgery: a controlled clinical trial. J Hand Surg Am 17:132–136.

88. Meyers SA, Seaber AV, Glisson RR, Nunley JA (1989) Effect of hyaluronic acid/chondroitin sulfate on healing of full-thickness tendon lacerations in rabbits. J Orthop Res 7:683–689.

89. Miller JA, Ferguson RL, Powers DL et al (1997) Efficacy of hyaluronic acid/nonsteroidal anti-inflammatory drug systems in preventing postsurgical tendon adhesions. J Biomed Mater Res 38:25–33.

90. Tzianabos AO, Cisneros RL, Gershkovich J et al (1999) Effect of surgical adhesion reduction devices on the propagation of experimental intra-abdominal infection. Archives of Surgery 134:1254–1259.

91. Murphy PG, Loitz BJ, Frank CB, Hart DA (1994) Influence of exogenous growth factors on the synthesis and secretion of collagen types I and III by explants of normal and healing rabbit ligaments. Biochemistry and Cell Biology 72:403–409.

92. Schmidt CC, Georgescu HI, Kwoh CK et al (1995) Effect of growth factors on the proliferation of fibroblasts from the medial collateral and anterior cruciate ligaments. J Orthop Res 13:184–190.

93. Spindler KP, Dawson JM, Stahlman GC et al (2002) Collagen expression and biomechanical response to human recombinant transforming growth factor beta (rhTGF-beta2) in the healing rabbit MCL. J Orthop Res 20:318–324.

94. Woo SL, Smith DW, Hildebrand KA et al (1998) Engineering the healing of the rabbit medial collateral ligament. Medical and Biological Engineering and Computing 36:359–364.

95. Letson AK, Dahners LE (1994) The effect of combinations of growth factors on ligament healing. Clin Orthop Relat Res 308:207–212.

96. Pierce GF, Mustoe TA, Lingelbach J et al (1989) Platelet-derived growth factor and transforming growth factor-beta enhance tissue repair activities by unique mechanisms. Journal of Cell Biology 109:429–440.

97. Kobayashi D, Kurosaka M, Yoshiya S, Mizuno K (1997) Effect of basic fibroblast growth factor on the healing of defects in the canine anterior cruciate ligament. [see comments.]. Knee Surgery, Sports Traumatology, Arthroscopy 5:189–194.

98. Hildebrand KA, Woo SL, Smith DW et al (1998) The effects of platelet-derived growth factor-BB on healing of the rabbit medial collateral ligament. An in vivo study. American Journal of Sports Medicine 26:549–554.

99. Robinson SN, Talmadge JE (2002) Sustained release of growth factors. In Vivo 16:535–540.

100. Edwards RB, 3rd, Seeherman HJ, Bogdanske JJ et al (2004) Percutaneous injection of recombinant human bone morphogenetic protein-2 in a calcium phosphate paste accelerates healing of a canine tibial osteotomy. J Bone Joint Surg Am 86-A:1425–1438.

101. Mercier NR, Constantino HR, Tracy MA, Bonassar LJ (2004) A novel injectable approach for cartilage formation in vivo using PLG microspheres. Annals of Biomedical Engineering 32:418–429.

102. Burdick JA, Mason MN, Hinman AD et al (2002) Delivery of osteoinductive growth factors from degradable PEG hydrogels influences osteoblast differentiation and mineralization. Journal of Controlled Release 83:53–63.

103. Lam XM, Duenas ET, Cleland JL (2001) Encapsulation and stabilization of nerve growth factor into poly(lactic-co-glycolic) acid microspheres. Journal of Pharmaceutical Sciences 90:1356–1365.

104. Azuma H, Yasuda K, Tohyama H et al (2003) Timing of administration of transforming growth factor-beta and epidermal growth factor influences the effect on material properties of the in situ frozen-thawed anterior cruciate ligament. J Biomech 36:373–381.

105. Tabata Y, Miyao M, Yamamoto M, Ikada Y (1999) Vascularization into a porous sponge by sustained release of basic fibroblast growth factor. Journal of Biomaterials Science. Polymer Edition 10:957–968.

106. Batten ML, Hansen JC, Dahners LE (1996) Influence of dosage and timing of application of platelet-derived growth factor on early healing of the rat medial collateral ligament. J Orthop Res 14:736–741.

107. Kawai K, Suzuki S, Tabata Y et al (2000) Accelerated tissue regeneration through incorporation of basic fibroblast growth factor-impregnated gelatin microspheres into artificial dermis. Biomaterials 21:489–499.

108. Downs EC, Robertson NE, Riss TL, Plunkett ML (1992) Calcium alginate beads as a slow-release system for delivering angiogenic molecules in vivo and in vitro. Journal of Cell Physiology 152:422–429.

109. Inui K, Maeda M, Sano A et al (1998) Local application of basic fibroblast growth factor minipellet induces the healing of segmental bony defects in rabbits. Calcif Tissue Int 63:490–495.

110. Kanematsu A, Yamamoto S, Noguchi T et al (2003) Bladder regeneration by bladder acellular matrix combined with sustained release of exogenous growth factor. Journal of Urology 170:1633–1638.

111. Lee AC, Yu VM, Lowe JB, 3rd, et al (2003) Controlled release of nerve growth factor enhances sciatic nerve regeneration. Experimental Neurology 184:295–303.

112. Murphy WL, Peters MC, Kohn DH, Mooney DJ (2000) Sustained release of vascular endothelial growth factor from mineralized poly(lactide-co-glycolide) scaffolds for tissue engineering. Biomaterials 21:2521–2527.

113. Tanihara M, Suzuki Y, Yamamoto E et al (2001) Sustained release of basic fibroblast growth factor and angiogenesis in a novel covalently crosslinked gel of heparin and alginate. J Biomed Mater Res 56:216–221.

114. Sakiyama-Elbert SE, Hubbell JA (2000) Development of fibrin derivatives for controlled release of heparin-binding growth factors. Journal of Controlled Release 65:389–402.

115. Sakiyama-Elbert SE, Hubbell JA (2000) Controlled release of nerve growth factor from a heparin-containing fibrin-based cell ingrowth matrix. Journal of Controlled Release 69:149–158.

116. Sakiyama-Elbert S, Das R, Gelberman RH et al (2008) Controlled release kinetics and biologic activity of PDGF-BB for use in flexor tendon repair. J Hand Surg Am 33:1548–1557.

117. Suzuki M, Asplund T, Yamashita H et al (1995) Stimulation of hyaluronan biosynthesis by platelet-derived growth factor-BB and transforming growth factor-beta 1 involves activation of protein kinase C. Biochemical Journal 307:817–821.

118. Bartold PM (1993) Platelet-derived growth factor stimulates hyaluronate but not proteoglycan synthesis by human gingival fibroblasts in vitro. Journal of Dental Research 72:1473–1480.

119. Heldin P, Pertoft H (1993) Synthesis and assembly of the hyaluronan-containing coats around normal human mesothelial cells. Experimental Cell Research 208:422–429.

120. Papakonstantinou E, Karakiulakis G, Roth M, Block LH (1995) Platelet-derived growth factor stimulates the secretion of hyaluronic acid by proliferating human vascular smooth muscle cells. Proceedings of the Nationall Academy of Sciences of the U S A 92:9881–9885.

121. Evanko SP, Johnson PY, Braun KR et al (2001) Platelet-derived growth factor stimulates the formation of versican-hyaluronan aggregates and pericellular matrix expansion in arterial smooth muscle cells. Archives of Biochemistry and Biophysics 394:29–38.

122. Pullen M, Thomas K, Wu H, Nambi P (2001) Stimulation of Hyaluronan synthetase by platelet-derived growth factor bb in human prostate smooth muscle cells. Pharmacology 62:103–106.

123. Dunlop ME, Clark S, Mahadevan P et al (1996) Production of hyaluronan by glomerular mesangial cells in response to fibronectin and platelet derived growth factor. Kidney International 50:40–44.
124. Tiedemann K, Malmstrom A, Westergren-Thorsson G (1997) Cytokine regulation of proteoglycan production in fibroblasts: separate and synergistic effects. Matrix Biology 15:469–478.
125. Asplund T, Versnel MA, Laurent TC, Heldin P (1993) Human mesothelioma cells produce factors that stimulate the production of hyaluronan by mesothelial cells and fibroblasts. Cancer Research 53:388–392.
126. Hamada Y, Katoh S, Hibino N et al (2006) Effects of monofilament nylon coated with basic fibroblast growth factor on endogenous intrasynovial flexor tendon healing. J Hand Surg Am 31:530–540.

Peripheral Nerve Regeneration by Artificial Nerve Guides

9

A. Merolli and L. Rocchi

Abstract It is more than 20 years since artificial nerve guides (or conduits) were introduced into clinical practice as a reliable alternative to autograft. They are basically cylindrical conduits inside which a regenerating nerve stump may find protection and guidance. Early guides were made of silicone and were not biodegradable; they were shown to support nerve regeneration but, subsequently, were considered responsible for stenosis of the regenerated nerve in several instances, which required their removal. Degradable guides have been proposed and are now widely used. An overview of the clinical outcome of artificial nerve guides in peripheral nerve-gap injuries has shown that they perform at least as well as autografts in gaps that are no longer than 20 mm, bringing the significant advantage of avoiding donor site sacrifice and morbidity. The present knowledge and limitations of contemporary nerve guides are illustrated; research to improve the present designs is discussed.

Keywords Artificial Nerve Guide • Biocompatible Glues • Nerve-gap Lesion • Nerve Regeneration • Nerve Suture

9.1
Introduction

The permanent damage and social costs of peripheral nerve injuries are increasingly unacceptable. The results of current therapies are not fully satisfactory and the rate of successful recovery from peripheral nerve lesions is far from being optimal despite progress in microsurgery [1–3]. Several variables are involved: age, for example, since the rate of unsuccessful recovery from peripheral nerve-gap lesions in the elderly is higher than average [1,4,5]; type of injury is also important, since sharp blade injuries with no gap between the stumps have a far better prognosis than avulsion injuries, with torn and crushed nerve tissue and a gap being produced later [5]; timing of treatment, because lesions that are not acutely treated have a worse prognosis. Unfortunately, the latter are not uncommon because of the frequent association of nerve injures with major polytrauma, which, sometimes, means they are neglected with a consequent delay to diagnosis or treatment.

A. Merolli (✉)
Orthopaedics and Hand Surgery, The Catholic University School of Medicine, Rome, Italy

A. Merolli, T.J. Joyce (eds), *Biomaterials in Hand Surgery.*
© Springer-Verlag Italia 2009

The gold standard in treating nerve-gap injuries is the autograft [6]. Nerve auto-grafts contain acutely denervated, "axon-responsive" Schwann cells, lying within a scaffold of longitudinally aligned basal laminae, and providing a microenvironment that facilitates axonal regrowth. Unfortunately, there are several limitations and complications associated with autografts, since harvesting a donor nerve graft may have significant co-morbidity [7–10]. Furthermore, the two stitch sutures (one proximal and one distal) required to secure the autograft may be the site where a possible occurrence of an unfavorable fibroblastic proliferation hinders progression of the tiny regenerating axons [11]. This will be particularly inconvenient for those regenerating axons that have succeeded in growing from the proximal stump, right along the graft, to the distal stump.

It is also possible that in future there will be increasing difficulty in proposing an autograft to patients, since they may not accept the sacrifice of another nerve in their body and the associated morbidity at the donor site, coupled with the lack of a guaranteed positive outcome of the grafting procedure. Additionally, they may perceive that, in the worst case, they will end up with two lesions instead of one.

It must also be considered that often the nerve at the donor site is a smaller sensitive nerve, and this limits full recovery from the outset, when a larger and more important motor nerve requires the treatment.

An alternative to autograft is allograft, which may bring even greater problems, such as the need for immunosuppressive control and therapy [5]. Recent commercial allografts claim to be non-immunogenic to the host; they are actually highly processed explanted nerves, provided in the form of cylinders that preserve the laminin-laden structure of the nerve fascicles [12]. In this construct they may be better assimilated to an artificial nerve guide than to a nerve with full integrity.

9.2
Tubular Nerve Guides

It is more than 20 years since artificial nerve guides (or conduits) were introduced into clinical practice as a reliable alternative to autograft (Fig. 9.1). They are basically cylindrical conduits inside which a regenerating nerve stump may find protection and guidance [13].

Early guides were made of silicone and were not biodegradable [14]; they were shown to support nerve regeneration but, subsequently, were considered responsible for stenosis of the regenerated nerve in several instances, which required their removal [15,16]. In sites such as, for example, the brachial plexus, the indication for mid-term removal of the guide, to avoid its stenosizing action, seemed inappropriate, and degradable guides were proposed.

An overview of the clinical outcome of artificial nerve guides in peripheral nerve gap injuries showed that they perform at least as well as autografts in gaps that are no longer than 20 mm, bringing the significant advantage of avoiding donor site sacrifice and morbidity [17,18]. Nowadays there are several degradable nerve guides in clinical

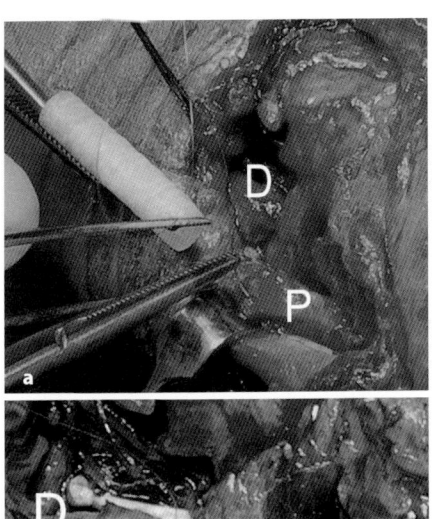
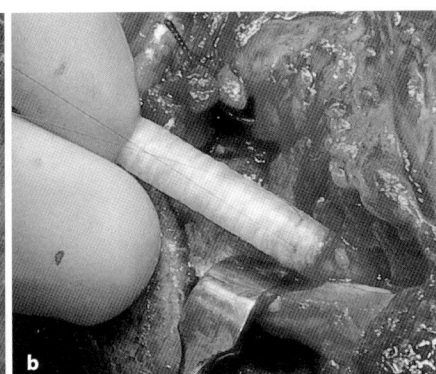
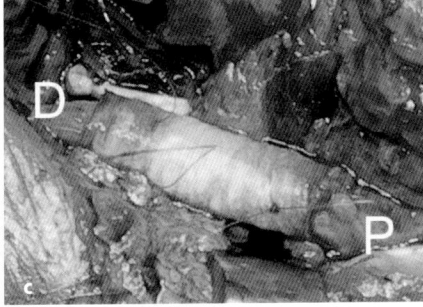

Fig. 9.1 A treated-collagen nerve guide has been used to bridge the trimmed stumps of a gap lesion in the ulnar nerve at the wrist. A loop was made from the guide to the proximal stump (P) (**a**), which was then gently accommodated inside the lumen (**b**); the same procedure was performed to accommodate the distal stump (D) (**c**)

use [19]; they are made of polyglycolic acid ("Neurotube" Synovis USA), poly-lactic-acid ("Neurolac" Ascension USA – Polyganics NL), and treated bovine collagen ("Neuragen" Integra USA; "Neuroflex" and "Neuromatrix" Stryker – Collagen Matrix USA). A proprietary hydrogel that is non-degradable *in vivo* has been used to produce a nerve guide ("SaluBridge" SaluMedica USA), and several other experimental guides have been proposed and tested *in vitro* and *in vivo* [20–57]. Apart from the length, the diameter of the lumen of the cylindrical conduit seems relevant in terms of a successful recovery [58]. This may be due to the possible occurrence of central areas of insufficient vascularization in guides or scaffolds with a larger lumen.

Many features are required of the nerve conduit to favor regeneration. It must direct axons sprouting from the proximal to the distal stump; it has to minimize fibroblast infiltration from the outside and, at the same time, retain a certain degree of porosity to allow cells to set and migrate inside the tube. The guide also needs to provide adequate mechanical strength and flexibility to support the regenerating nerve fibers and, obviously, must be biocompatible.

Several studies have been published on nerve guides, and several research studies on the topic of nerve regeneration by artificial nerve guides are currently in progress [59]. An extensive literature suggests that they must include the provision of a biocompatible and bioresorbable scaffold that is able to support outgrowing axons and their associated cells, and within which the microenvironment of a peripheral nerve fiber can be replicated. With an artificial nerve guide, axonal regeneration may occur along longitudinal structures, guiding the nerve, in the presence of neurotrophic and neurotropic factors, which can either be added locally or concentrated in the chamber constituted by the conduit; the presence of viable Schwann cells could be essential. Nanotechnology has been advocated, by means of photolithographic and microprinting techniques that could be used to make patterns of organofunctional groups [60].

However, most of the guides in current use are basically empty and unstructured.

From the biomaterial point of view, the structural components of a nerve guide can be grouped into three parts (Fig. 9.2): the outer structure, which is basically the tube inside which the nerve stumps are accommodated; the inner structure, which is how the tube is filled; and the suture: this last part seems to be seldom considered but it is the site where mechanical force is applied to the guide and mechanical and biological insult are imposed on the nerve stump.

A survey of the literature shows several proposals for each of the three parts, but there is little agreement among experimental results or opinions relating to the design for each of them.

The outer structure of the guide has been proposed as impermeable or selectively permeable to molecules but not cells, or permeable to cells as well. It has been proposed as rigid or flexible, degradable or non-degradable.

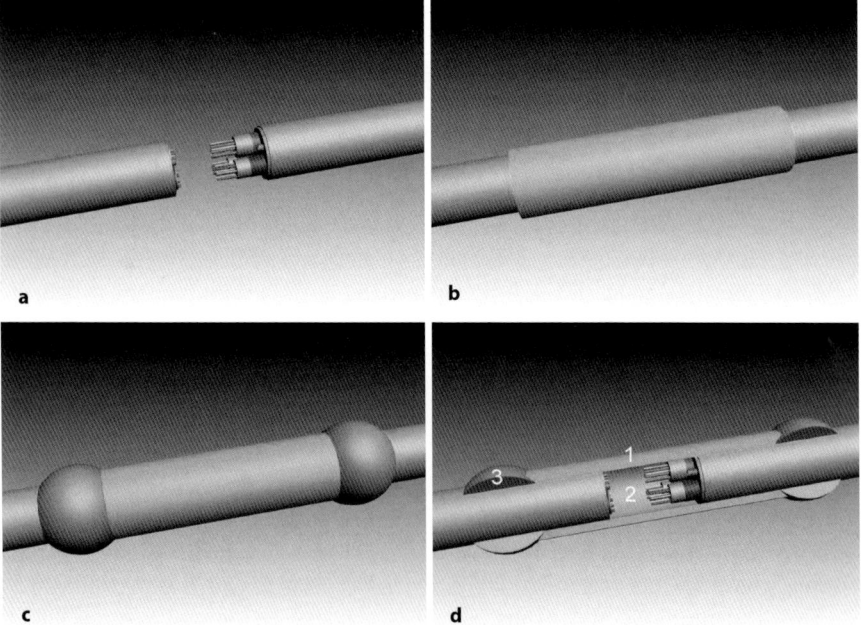

Fig. 9.2 Modeling a nerve gap lesion (**a**) treated by a cylindrical nerve guide (**b**) and secured by two drops of glue (**c**) helps to highlight the three parts (**d**) into which biomaterial research is focused: (*1*) the outer structure; (*2*) the inner structure; (*3*) the suture

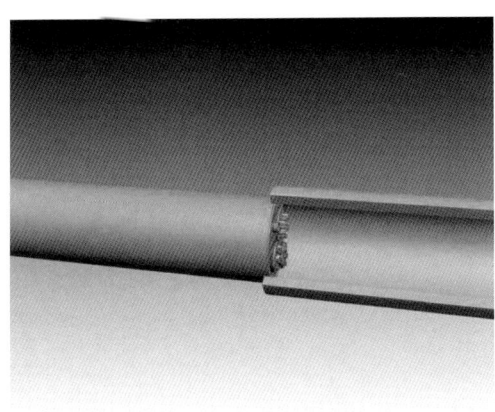

Fig. 9.3 From a surgical point of view, it may not be easy to accommodate a nerve stump inside a cylindrical guide of suitable diameter without manipulating it, sometimes heavily

The inner structure has been proposed as basically absent, being constituted by saline solution only, or highly structured, for example by the filling of longitudinal degradable fibers, or being able to deliver growth factors in a controlled way, or resembling the outer structure of the nerve fascicles.

The suture part has seen the use of several combinations of stitches and various options to accommodate the stumps, and of different types of glues. This interface between the guide and the nerve has received minor attention until now, but it is a very crucial point both surgically and biologically.

From a surgical point of view, it is not easy to accommodate a nerve stump inside a cylindrical guide of suitable diameter without manipulating it (sometimes heavily) and, anyway, stitch suture is still the most recommended method to hold the guide in place (Fig. 9.3). From a biological point of view, excessive manipulation of an already suffering nerve stump should be avoided, and stitch suture is a well-known cause of local inflammatory response. Fibrin glue has been used, with or without the association of stitch sutures. Glue, of any kind, is not easy to apply in a real surgical setting where the presence of blood and other fluids is highly variable.

9.3
Glue versus Stitches

A critical point that must be addressed is the need to use biocompatible glues in the substitution of microsutures (stitches). Established surgical treatment in sharp blade acute transection of a peripheral nerve, with negligible or absent gap, prescribes the joining of the two stumps by an end-to-end suture (neurorraphy) [61]. It is widely accepted that the suture should not put the two stumps under tensional stress [62], because this will greatly favor the development of a fibroblastic and myofibroblastic proliferation. This phenomenon, whatever the cause, will impair and eventually stop any axonal regeneration [63]. But even without tensioning the stumps, it is the use of

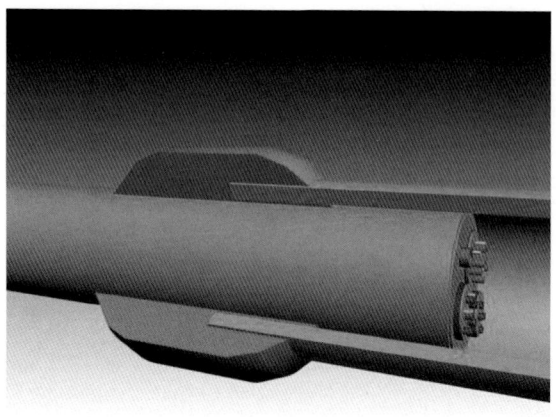

Fig. 9.4 The setting of the glue should be not too fast, to give the surgeon adequate time to accurately put the stumps in place, but should not be too slow, to avoid the accidental flow of part of the glue in front of the stump with the consequence of sealing it

stitches for the suture (both degradable and non-degradable) that promotes fibroblastic and myofibroblastic proliferation and may provoke sufficient inflammatory reaction and fibrosis to impair nerve regeneration, resulting in the same complications as already described [11]. Fibroblastic and myofibroblastic proliferation, and the eventual retraction of the surgical scar, are among the most adverse events against nerve fiber regeneration; they are not easily avoidable but, on the other hand, they should not be favored by using stitches to make the suture. In view of this, the use of sutures should be abandoned in favor of biocompatible glues in any surgery associated with neural structures and artificial nerve guides. Unfortunately, knowledge about glues is limited. There are promising results with cyanoacrylate molecules, and findings published in the literature show that cyanoacrylate glues can be used in direct contact with the nerve [64–68]. However, the use of glue in a true surgical setting still presents many unresolved problems. In principle, it is not easy to control the setting of the glue, which should be not too fast, to give the surgeon adequate time to accurately put the stumps in place, but should not be too slow, to avoid accidental flow of part of the glue in front of the stump with the consequence of sealing it (Fig. 9.4). Also, the method of glue application in a real surgical environment may be a problem. For example, some biphasic glues that may have suitable characteristics, when used in the tiny quantities required by a digital nerve suture, could polymerize early inside the microscopic delivery tube. Furthermore, unpredictable bleeding may eliminate the effectiveness of a gluing procedure if nerve surgery is performed with limited or absent intraoperative ischemia (tourniquet), as advocated to better preserve the delicate vascularization of the nerve.

9.4
Control Macromolecules and Seeded Cells

Research has also focused on the importance of cellular functions and inflammatory mechanisms, since recovery can be improved by altering cellular responses immediately after injury. Axonal regeneration from the neural cell could be accomplished more easily if the cascade of inflammatory and immunological events associated with the injury could be better controlled and maybe re-oriented. Methylprednisolone appears to reduce the damage to the nerve cells and to decrease inflammation near the injury site by suppressing activities of immune cells. Although cytokines can be toxic to nerve cells because they stimulate the production of free radicals, nitric oxide, and other inflammatory substances that cause cell death, they also stimulate the production of neurotrophic factors, which are beneficial to cell repair. Several types of cells have been studied for their potential to promote regeneration and repair, including Schwann cells, olfactory ensheathing glia, fetal spinal cord cells, and embryonic stem cells. Schwann cells, possibly harvested from the recipient, cultured, and deposited in an artificial nerve guide could be a key element in successful regeneration.

In any case, it is important to stress that to achieve the goal of regeneration, it is not sufficient to deliver growth factors to injured neurons, since they appear to encourage sprouting more than they stimulate regeneration for long distances. So, a kind of physical guidance may be necessary in the form of a specific surface topography [69]. Whether topography alone will suffice in guiding nerve regeneration has still to be proved [70], but it is possible that adequate topography, coupled with seeding of a gradient of control macromolecules delivered at the proper time, will be the key to success.

9.5
Clinical Limitations of the Tubular Nerve Guides

There are some limitations in the clinical application of commercially available tubular nerve guides. First, the tubular structure in itself makes surgical implantation difficult, because a precise diameter matching between the guide and the nerve is not always possible and, furthermore, while a larger guide should be implanted at the start, to favor minimum damage in entering the nerve stump, during healing the nerve can grow larger and the guide can stenotize the regenerated nerve, even when a bioresorbable material has been used to manufacture it [71]. Secondly, stitch sutures are required to secure commercially available guides. Even if they may be restricted to a minimum of one per side, they represent a site where unfavorable fibroblastic reaction may ensue. Thirdly, greater length and greater diameter of the guide reduce the success of nerve regeneration. This may be partly due to the occurrence of a central area of poorer vascularization.

Perhaps it is the concurrent action of these factors that sums up the most important limitation of tubular nerve guides, from the clinical point of view: so far none of the options available has performed satisfactorily in bridging gaps longer than 30 mm.

Another debatable point is the need to avoid intraoperative ischemia while operating on a peripheral nerve. It seems that avoiding the tourniquet reduces the damage to the tiny nerve fibers. Critical damage may be associated with: (1) temporary hypoxia; (2) mechanical insult due to blood overflow following tourniquet release; (3) a possible rise in the concentration of catabolic factors produced and accumulated during temporary ischemia; and (4) blood clotting.

On the other hand, it is difficult to envisage surgery without a tourniquet in complex trauma of the limbs, and in several other clinical scenarios where lesions to nerves are not the only damage.

9.6
The Role of Intraneural Vascularization in Defining the Effectiveness of Nerve Regeneration

The nerve's vascular supply is made up of an intricate network of increasingly smaller vessels all around the epineurium and perineurium and, finally, dispersed among individual nerve fibers inside each fascicle (Fig. 9.5).

A common law seems to apply any time artificial regeneration of a living tissue is attempted: effective regeneration must include the concurrent development of a proper vascular supply. Several studies have examined the possibility of stimulating or directing angiogenesis along the artificial regenerative process under study. However, another perspective may suggest that correct tissue regeneration implies that a proper angiogenesis has been achieved in parallel.

In the specific task of peripheral nerve regeneration, most studies focus on the best possible distribution of regenerated nerve fibers to resemble that of an intact nerve. As already stated, regeneration over distances longer than 20–30 mm, or for nerves of large diameters, is still a challenge, and a careful look at the intraneural vascularization is not always highlighted. Successful nerve regeneration should probably be defined concurrently with assessment of an adequate, newly formed, vascular supply. It is known that after injury, neurons redirect their metabolism towards the regeneration of new axons, while Schwann cells replicate and try to match and nurture them.

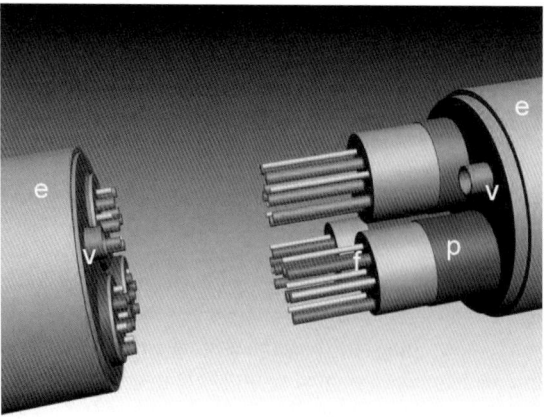

Fig. 9.5 While modeling a peripheral nerve with its ensheathing epineurium (*e*), the perineurium (*p*) which delimits each fascicle, and the myelinated and non-myelinated nerve fibers (*f*) inside each fascicle, it is important not to forget the constant presence of blood vessels (*v*)

However, even with the adequate protection and guidance of the artificial environment of a suitably engineered nerve guide, we should ask the question: how far can nerve regeneration proceed without an adequate vascular support? In addition: does the key to successful nerve regeneration lie in promoting intraneural vascularization as well as axonal elongation?

9.7
The NeuroBox Concept and the Search for a Nerve Regeneration Technique that is Surgically Easier, Biologically Respectful, and Technologically Affordable

In 2006, authors developed and tested *in vivo* a new concept of nerve guide which is double-halved, non-degradable, and rigid, and does not require the use of any stitch sutured to the nerve stump, allowing the use of cyanoacrylic glue instead (Fig. 9.6).

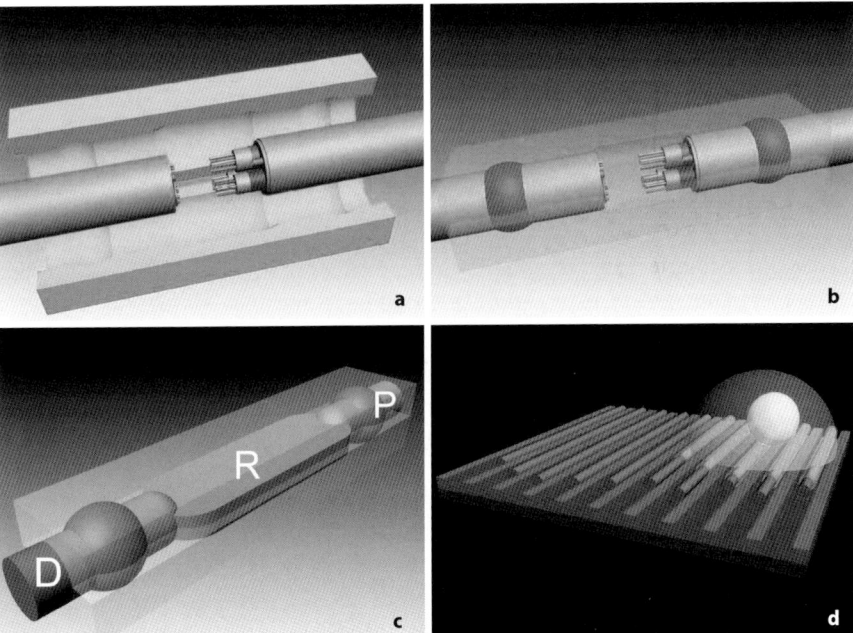

Fig. 9.6 The NeuroBox concept replaces the traditional cylindrical nerve guide by a box of two halves (**a**), into which the neural stumps are accommodated and glued in a dedicated compartment (**b**); elongating axons grow inside a flat "regeneration chamber" (*R*), placed between the proximal (*P*) and distal (*D*) nerve stumps (**c**) and whose floor is paved by a microstructure called the "carpet", where trenches 1.5 μm deep and 10 μm wide have been microcarved along the longitudinal axis. These trenches are aimed at homing regenerating axons with the protective coverage of Schwann's cells (**d**)

In the NeuroBox, the traditional cylindrical nerve guide is replaced by a box of two halves in which three main compartments are recognizable: (1) a lodgement for the neural stump (one proximal and one distal); (2) a compartment for the acrylate glue (one proximal and one distal); and (3) a flat "regeneration chamber" of 4.0 x 3.5 x 2.0 mm (length x width x height).

The dedicated glue compartment of the NeuroBox promotes polymerization of the glue with the minimum amount that is needed to wet it; neural stumps are gently accommodated within their compartments prior to the end of the polymerization process.

The key element of the NeuroBox is the flat "regeneration chamber": in this compartment, the bunch of fibers of the proximal stump is invited to spread on a wider flat surface. The chamber can receive several treatments like the micro- and nanocarving of dedicated topography; the implantation of molecules that may enhance nerve growth and inhibit fibroblastic proliferation; the accommodation of scaffolds; and the seeding of cells.

A structure called the "carpet" is glued to the floor. The "carpet" is a 4.5 x 3 mm sheet of polymethyl-methacrylate (PMMA), with trenches 1.5 µm deep and 10 µm wide, microcarved along the longitudinal axis. These trenches are aimed at homing regenerating axons with the protective coverage of Schwann's cells. The guide cannot be considered completely sealed but, on the contrary, some empty space remains at both entrances. Fluids such as irrigation saline fluid, and cells may access the chamber.

In an experimental study in a rat sciatic nerve model [72], nerve regeneration occurred in all animals treated by the implantation of the NeuroBox (Fig. 9.7). In regenerated nerves, at retrieval, a yellowish cord joined the two stumps, presenting a fine blood vessel network at its periphery. The retrieved nerve was longer than the contralateral intact nerve.

When multiple *in vivo* inspections took place, at 7 days, a yellowish material, and what seemed to be a reddish clot, contoured the access to the regeneration chamber at both ends, while the chamber itself remained substantially empty. At 20 days, a yellowish material spanned between the two stumps, and red stripes and spots were associated with it. At 34 days the yellowish material had formed a cylindrical cord, and a fine vascular network was observed at its periphery. At 63 days a regenerated nerve was retrieved. A fibrous capsule was found around the guide but not inside the regeneration chamber.

In visible light microscopy, the regenerated zone showed large and small fibers whose myelin sheath was less thick, as expected in the case of an ongoing myelinization process, but there was more abundant cellularity among the fibers. Transmission electron microscopy allowed identification of several myelinated axons undergoing the myelinization process but also several non-myelinated fibers with mitochondria embraced by the cytoplasm of Schwann's cells. Fine blood vessels were well represented. There were no signs of intraneural fibrosis or other adverse intraneural reactions.

In the distal end zone, tiny myelinated and non-myelinated fibers were present, evidencing regenerated axons that entered the distal stump. In the proximal and distal glueing end zones, the outer fibroelastic sheath that was in direct contact with the glue showed no major alterations.

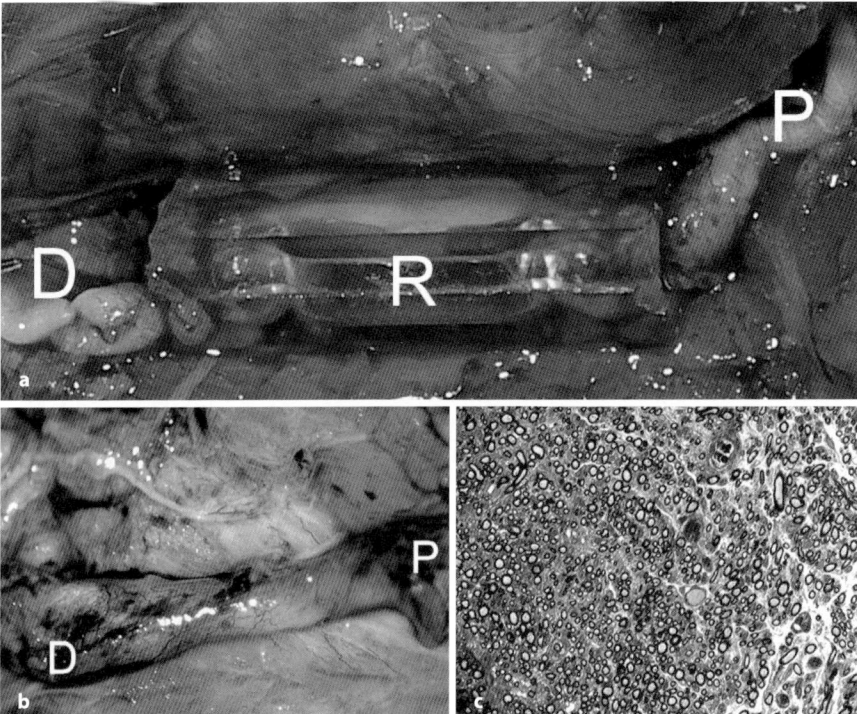

Fig. 9.7 Nerve regeneration occurred in a NeuroBox implanted in a rat sciatic nerve gap lesion (**a**). The newly formed nerve regenerate joins the proximal and the distal stumps after 2 months (**b**). In visible light microscopy the regenerated zone showed large and small fibers whose myelin sheath was less thick than the contralateral intact nerve, as expected in the case of an ongoing myelinization process, but there is more abundant cellularity among the fibers (**c**). *D*, distal; *P*, proximal; *R*, regenerating portion

The concept of the box may help with surgical implantation of the guide. It is easier to accommodate the nerve stumps inside the half-box without any of the damage that is possible, on the other hand, while trying to push/pull the nerve stump into a tailored diameter-matched tubular guide. The use of stitches may be abandoned since the stumps will be held in place by a glue cast around the nerve. Only a small range of sizes is needed for a surgical set, since the glue cast and flat regeneration chamber will help in adapting stumps of different diameters to the same guide.

A rigid guide, in principle, can provide better mechanical protection to the tiny fragile regenerating axons; however, from a clinical point of view, it is possible to envisage that there will be applications where a rigid guide may be preferable (for example, along the shaft of long bones) while there will be other applications where a flexible guide would be desirable (for example, close to a finger joint).

Tiny vessels found dispersed into the regenerated nerve may also support the speculation that the flat regeneration chamber can promote a better vascularization of the regenerated tissue, favoring the development of both a neural and a vessel network that should occur *in vivo* [73,74].

A lot of work has been done (and is ongoing) regarding topography *in vitro* (both micro- and nanotopography; in two- or three-dimensional scaffolds; with or without the implantation of macromolecules) [60,75–79]; this NeuroBox guide has facilitated an easy method of testing these parameters *in vivo*, since, in its regeneration chamber, in principle it reproduces a small *in vitro* system for axonal regeneration without the usual limitations of an *in vitro* experiment regarding translation of its results into the real *in vivo* situation.

9.8
Longer Gaps as a Current Challenge and Regeneration in the Absence of the Distal Stump as the Ultimate Challenge

Nerve regeneration over distances greater than 20 or 30 mm is the current challenge in both research and clinical application. Several parameters are involved and several current research studies are trying to promote longer-distance growth with the assistance of growth factors, dedicated topographies, and support cells. In both the laboratory and the clinic, the task to be accomplished is the final functional union between the proximal and the distal stumps of the injured nerve. Most of the artificial nerve guides already tested are effective in the presence of the distal stump and for shorter gaps.

However, regeneration in longer gaps may require a different approach, such as for the concept of a "dead-ended" nerve guide [36], namely a long guide where the proximal stump of the donor nerve is left to grow freely, with the sole assistance of the artificial device and its engineered structure (Fig. 9.8).

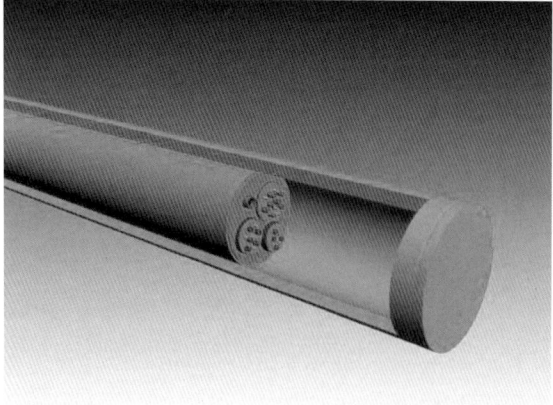

Fig. 9.8 In a "dead-ended" nerve guide, the proximal stump of the nerve is left to grow freely, with the sole assistance of the artificial device and its engineered structure

A huge potential application lies in the eventual discovery of an effective method to promote and control nerve regeneration in the absence of the distal stump, because this seems to be the most challenging clinical situations and, is unfortunately, a frequent occurrence.

Patients may lack a distal stump because, for example, they received treatment after a period longer than 3 months from trauma. However, another reason for nerve growth in the absence of the distal stump may be the situation when a very long gap is present which would require an excessive sacrifice of donor site for a graft and, then, would discourage nerve grafting procedures. Gaps longer than 100 mm, even in the presence of a distal stump, would probably benefit from the same technology of nerve regeneration in the absence of the distal stump.

A new perspective for this very long-distance growth in a "dead-ended" nerve guide may be the possibility of joining the central nervous system (CNS) to distal targets in patients with spinal cord injuries. It is difficult to predict if this will ever become a realistic option, but the discovery from Brunelli that a direct connection between the CNS and peripheral muscles does work, not only in laboratory animals [80,81] but also in humans [82], stimulates research into the artificial regeneration of nerves over very long distances, to overcome the need to graft extremely long segments of autologous nerves.

Note: the NeuroBox is an international patent of the Catholic University in Rome (WO/2008/029373).

References

1. Wolford LM, Stevao ELL (2003) Consideration in nerve repair. Proc (Bayl Univ Med Cent) 16:152–156.
2. Trumble TE, Archibald S, Allan CH (2004) Bioengineering for nerve repair in the future. J Am Soc Surg Hand 4:134–142.
3. Lundborg G, Rosen B (2007) Hand function after nerve repair. Acta Physiol 189:207–217.
4. Verdu E, Ceballos D, Vilches JJ, Navarro X (2000) Influence of aging on peripheral nerve function and regeneration. J Peripher Nerv Syst 5:191–208.
5. Dahlin LB (2008) Nerve injuries. Curr Orthop 22:9–16.
6. Sinis N, Schaller HE, Schulte-Eversum C et al (2007) Comparative neuro tissue engineering using different nerve guide implants. Acta Neurochir Suppl 100:61–64.
7. Staniforth P, Fisher TR (1978) The effects of sural nerve excision in autogenous nerve grafting. Hand 10:187–190.
8. Oritguela ME, Wood MB, Cahill D (1987) Anatomy of the sural nerve complex. J Hand Surg [Am] 12:1119–1123
9. Rappaport WD, Valente J, Hunter G (1993) Clinical utilization and complications of sural nerve biopsy. Am J Surg 166:252–256.
10. Taras JS, Nanavati V, Steelman P (2005) Nerve conduits. J Hand Ther 18:191–197.
11. Bora FW Jr (1967) Peripheral nerve repair in cats. The fascicular stitch. J Bone Joint Surg Am 49:659–666.
12. Neubauer D, Graham JB, Muir D (2007) Chondroitinase treatment increases the effective length of acellular nerve grafts. Exp Neurol 207:163–170.

13. Ijkema-Paassen J, Jansen K, Gramsbergen A, Meek MF (2004) Transection of peripheral nerves, bridging strategies and effect evaluation. Biomaterials 25:1583–1592.
14. Lundborg G, Dahlin LB, Danielsen N (1991) Ulnar nerve repair by the silicone chamber technique. Case report. Scand J Plast Reconstr Surg Hand Surg 25:79–82.
15. Merle M, Dellon AL, Campbell JN, Chang PS (1989) Complications from silicon-polymer intubulation of nerves. Microsurgery 10:130–133.
16. Dellon AL (1994) Use of a silicone tube for the reconstruction of a nerve injury. J Hand Surg [Br] 19:271–272.
17. Sinis N, Schaller HE, Schulte-Eversum C, Schlosshauer B et al (2005) Nerve regeneration across a 2-cm gap in the rat median nerve using a resorbable nerve conduit filled with Schwann cells. J Neurosurg 103:1067–1076.
18. Schlosshauer B, Dreesmann L, Schaller HE, Sinis N (2006) Synthetic nerve guide implants in humans: a comprehensive survey. Neurosurgery 59:740–747.
19. Meek MF, Coert JH (2008) US Food and Drug Administration/Conformit Europe-approved absorbable nerve conduits for clinical repair of peripheral and cranial nerves. Ann Plast Surg 60:110–116.
20. Ahmed MR, Vairamuthu S, Shafiuzama M et al (2005) Microwave irradiated collagen tubes as a better matrix for peripheral nerve regeneration. Brain Res 1046:55–67.
21. Bertleff MJ, Meek MF, Nicolai JP (2005) A prospective clinical evaluation of biodegradable neurolac nerve guides for sensory nerve repair in the hand. J Hand Surg [Am] 30:513–518.
22. Bozkurt A, Brook GA, Moellers S et al (2007) In vitro assessment of axonal growth using dorsal root ganglia explants in a novel three-dimensional collagen matrix. Tissue Eng 13:2971–2979.
23. Bunting S, Di Silvio L, Deb S, Hall S (2005) Bioresorbable glass fibres facilitate peripheral nerve regeneration. J Hand Surg [Br] 30:242–247.
24. Ceballos D, Navarro X, Dubey N et al (1999) Magnetically aligned collagen gel filling a collagen nerve guide improves peripheral nerve regeneration. Exp Neurol 158:290–300.
25. Chang CJ, Hsu SH, Yen HJ et al (2007) Effects of unidirectional permeability in asymmetric poly(DL-lactic acid-co-glycolic acid) conduits on peripheral nerve regeneration: an in vitro and in vivo study. J Biomed Mater Res B Appl Biomater 83:206–215.
26. Chang JY, Lin JH, Yao CH et al (2007) In vivo evaluation of a biodegradable EDC/NHS-cross-linked gelatin peripheral nerve guide conduit material. Macromol Biosci 7:500–507.
27. Chavez-Delgado ME, Gomez-Pinedo U, Feria-Velasco A et al (2005) Ultrastructural analysis of guided nerve regeneration using progesterone- and pregnenolone-loaded chitosan prostheses. J Biomed Mater Res B Appl Biomater 74:589–600.
28. Chen YS, Chang JY, Cheng CY et al (2005) An in vivo evaluation of a biodegradable genipin-cross-linked gelatin peripheral nerve guide conduit material. Biomaterials 26:3911–3918.
29. Ciardelli G, Chiono V (2006) Materials for peripheral nerve regeneration. Macromol Biosci 6:13–26.
30. Den Dunnen WF, van der Lei B, Robinson PH et al (1995) Biological performance of a degradable poly(lactic acid-epsilon-caprolactone) nerve guide: influence of tube dimensions. J Biomed Mater Res 29:757–766.
31. Den Dunnen WF, Stokroos I, Blaauw EH et al (1996) Light-microscopic and electron-microscopic evaluation of short-term nerve regeneration using a biodegradable poly(DL-lactide-epsilon-caprolacton) nerve guide. J Biomed Mater Res 31:105–115.
32. Gamez E, Goto Y, Nagata K et al (2004) Photofabricated gelatin-based nerve conduits: nerve tissue regeneration potentials. Cell Transplant 13:549–564.
33. Huang YC, Huang YY, Huang CC, Liu HC (2005) Manufacture of porous polymer nerve conduits through a lyophilizing and wire-heating process. J Biomed Mater Res B Appl Biomater 74:659–664.
34. Inada Y, Hosoi H, Yamashita A et al (2007) Regeneration of peripheral motor nerve gaps with

a polyglycolic acid-collagen tube: technical case report. Neurosurgery 61:E1105–1107.

35. Jansen K, Meek MF, van der Werff JF et al (2006) Long-term regeneration of the rat sciatic nerve through a biodegradable poly(DL-lactide-epsilon-caprolactone) nerve guide: tissue reactions with focus on collagen III/IV reformation. J Biomed Mater Res A 69:334–341.

36. Lewin-Kowalik J, Marcol W, Kotulska-Wolwender K et al (2003) Dead-ended autologous connective tissue chambers in peripheral nerve repair – early observations. Acta Physiol Hung 90:157–166.

37. Lietz M, Ullrich A, Schulte-Eversum C et al (2006) Physical and biological performance of a novel block copolymer nerve guide. Biotechnol Bioeng 93:99–109.

38. Lietz M, Dreesmann L, Hoss M et al (2006) Neuro tissue engineering of glial nerve guides and the impact of different cell types. Biomaterials 27:1425–1436.

39. Madaghiele M, Sannino A, Yannas IV, Spector M (2008) Collagen-based matrices with axially oriented pores. J Biomed Mater Res A 85:757–767.

40. Madison RD, da Silva C, Dikkes P et al (1987) Peripheral nerve regeneration with entubulation repair: comparison of biodegradeable nerve guides versus polyethylene tubes and the effects of a laminin-containing gel. Exp Neurol 95:378–390.

41. Marchesi C, Pluderi M, Colleoni F et al (2007) Skin-derived stem cells transplanted into resorbable guides provide functional nerve regeneration after sciatic nerve resection. Glia 55:425–438.

42. Nakamura T, Inada Y, Fukuda S et al (2004) Experimental study on the regeneration of peripheral nerve gaps through a polyglycolic acid-collagen (PGA-collagen) tube. Brain Res 1027:18–29.

43. Navarro X, Rodriguez FJ, Labrador RO et al (1996) Peripheral nerve regeneration through bioresorbable and durable nerve guides. J Peripher Nerv Syst 1:53–64.

44. Nicoli Aldini N, Fini M, Rocca M et al (2000) Guided regeneration with resorbable conduits in experimental peripheral nerve injuries. Int Orthop 24:121–125.

45. Oh SH, Lee JH (2007) Fabrication and characterization of hydrophilized porous PLGA nerve guide conduits by a modified immersion precipitation method. J Biomed Mater Res A 80:530–538.

46. Patel M, Vandevord PJ, Matthew II et al (2006) Video-gait analysis of functional recovery of nerve repaired with chitosan nerve guides. Tissue Eng 12:3189–3199.

47. Patel M, Mao L, Wu B, Vandevord PJ (2007) GDNF-chitosan blended nerve guides: a functional study. J Tissue Eng Regen Med 1:360–367.

48. Pereira Lopes FR, Camargo de Moura Campos L, Dias Corrêa J Jr et al (2006) Bone marrow stromal cells and resorbable collagen guidance tubes enhance sciatic nerve regeneration in mice. Exp Neurol 198:457–468.

49. Phillips JB, Bunting SC, Hall SM, Brown RA (2005) Neural tissue engineering: a self-organizing collagen guidance conduit. Tissue Eng 11:1611–1617.

50. Scherman P, Kanje M, Dahlin LB (2005) Sutures as longitudinal guides for the repair of nerve defects – influence of suture numbers and reconstruction of nerve bifurcations. Restor Neurol Neurosci 23:79–85.

51. Stokols S, Tuszynski MH (2006) Freeze-dried agarose scaffolds with uniaxial channels stimulate and guide linear axonal growth following spinal cord injury. Biomaterials 27:443–451.

52. Stokols S, Sakamoto J, Breckon C et al (2006) Templated agarose scaffolds support linear axonal regeneration. Tissue Eng 12:2777–2787.

53. Sundback CA, Shyu JY, Wang Y et al (2005) Biocompatibility analysis of poly(glycerol sebacate) as a nerve guide material. Biomaterials 26:5454–5464.

54. Tos P, Battiston B, Nicolino S et al (2007) Comparison of fresh and predegenerated muscle-vein-combined guides for the repair of rat median nerve. Microsurgery 27:48–55.

55. Tyner TR, Parks N, Faria S et al (2007) Effects of collagen nerve guide on neuroma formation and neuropathic pain in a rat model. Am J Surg 193:e1–6.

56. Uebersax L, Mattotti M, Papaloizos M et al (2007) Silk fibroin matrices for the controlled release of nerve growth factor (NGF). Biomaterials 28:4449–4460.

57. Yoshitani M, Fukuda S, Itoi S et al (2007) Experimental repair of phrenic nerve using a polyglycolic acid and collagen tube. J Thorac Cardiovasc Surg 133:726–732.

58. Stang F, Fansa H, Wolf G, Reppin M, Keilhoff G (2005) Structural parameters of collagen nerve grafts influence peripheral nerve regeneration. Biomaterials 26:3083–3091.

59. Pfister LA, Papaloizos M, Merkle HP, Gander B (2007) Nerve conduits and growth factor delivery in peripheral nerve repair. J Peripher Nerv Syst 12:65–82.

60. Corey JM, Feldman EL (2003) Substrate patterning: an emerging technology for the study of neuronal behavior. Exp Neurol 184(Suppl 1):S89–96.

61. Millesi H (1981) Reappraisal of nerve repair. Surg Clin North Am 61:321–340.

62. Millesi H, Meissl G, Berger A (1976) Further experience with interfascicular grafting of the median, ulnar and radial nerves. J Bone Joint Surg Am 58:209–218.

63. Yannas IV, Zhang M, Spilker MH (2007) Standardized criterion to analyze and directly compare various materials and models for periphral nerve regeneration. J Biomater Sci Polym Ed 18:943–966.

64. Choi BH, Kim BY, Huh JY et al (2004) Microneural anastomosis using cyanoacrylate adhesives. Int J Oral Maxillofac Surg 33(8):777–780.

65. Piñeros-Fernández A, Rodeheaver PF, Rodeheaver GT (2005) Octyl 2-cyanoacrylate for repair of peripheral nerve. Ann Plast Surg 55:188–195.

66. Landegren T, Risling M, Brage A, Persson JK (2006) Long-term results of peripheral nerve repair: a comparison of nerve anastomosis with ethyl-cyanoacrylate and epineural sutures. Scand J Plast Reconstr Surg Hand Surg 40:65–72.

67. Elgazzar RF, Abdulmajeed I, Mutabbakani M (2007) Cyanoacrylate glue versus suture in peripheral nerve reanastomosis. Oral Surg Oral Med Oral Pathol Oral Radiol Endod 104:465–472.

68. Rickett T, Li J, Patel M, Sun W (2008) Ethyl-cyanoacrylate is acutely nontoxic and provides sufficient bond strength for anastomosis of peripheral nerves. J Biomed Mater Res A 20 Jun epub ahead of print.

69. Luckenbill-Edds L (1997) Laminin and the mechanism of neuronal outgrowth; Brain Res Brain Res Rev 23:1–27.

70. Liuzzi FJ, Tedeschi B (1991) Peripheral nerve regeneration; Neurosurg Clin N Am 2:31–42.

71. Merolli A, Rocchi L, Catalano F (2009) Ulnar nerve regeneration in a 70-years-old patient assessed upon revision of a degradable nerve-guide after nine months. J Reconstruc Microsurg 25(4):279–281

72. Merolli A, Rocchi L, Catalano F et al (2009) In-vivo regeneration of rat sciatic nerve in a double-halved stitch-less guide: a pilot-study. Microsurgery 29(4):310–318

73. Eichmann A, Le Noble F, Autiero M, Carmeliet P (2005) Guidance of vascular and neural network formation. Curr Opin Neurobiol 15:108–115.

74. Weinstein BM (2005) Vessels and nerves: marching to the same tune. Cell 120:299–302.

75. Kalil K, Dent EW (2005) Touch and go: guidance cues signal to the growth cone cytoskeleton. Curr Opin Neurobiol 15:521–526.

76. Michler A, Meyer DL (1989) Contact-guidance of neurite growth: a direct or an indirect effect of physical environment? J Hirnforsch 30:473–477.

77. Niere M, Braun B, Gass R et al (2006) Combination of engineered neural cell adhesion molecules and GDF-5 for improved neurite extension in nerve guide concepts. Biomaterials 27:3432–3440.

78. Rosner BI, Siegel RA, Grosberg A, Tranquillo RT (2003) Rational design of contact guiding, neurotrophic matrices for peripheral nerve regeneration. Ann Biomed Eng 31:1383–1401.

79. Thompson DM, Buettner HM (2006) Neurite outgrowth is directed by schwann cell alignment in the absence of other guidance cues. Ann Biomed Eng 34:161–168.

80. Brunelli G, Milanesi S (1988) Experimental repair of spinal cord lesions by grafting from CNS to PNS. J Reconstr Microsurg 4:245–50.
81. Brunelli GA, Brunelli GR (1996) Experimental surgery in spinal cord lesions by connecting upper motoneurons directly to peripheral targets. J Peripher Nerv Syst 1:111–118.
82. Brunelli G, Wild K (2008) Unsuspected plasticity of single neurons after connection of the corticospinal tract with peripheral nerves in spinal cord lesions. J Reconstr Microsurg 24:301–304.

Printed in July 2009